Department of Veterans Affairs
Health Services Research & Development Service | Evidence-based Synthesis Program

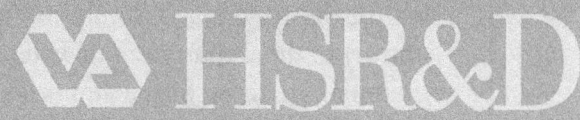

I0470875

Determining Key Features of Effective Depression Interventions

March 2009

Prepared for:

Department of Veterans Affairs
Veterans Health Administration
Health Services Research
& Development Service
Washington, DC 20420

Prepared by:

Greater Los Angeles Veterans Affairs Healthcare
System/Southern California/RAND
Evidence-based Practice Center
Los Angeles, CA

Investigators

Lisa V. Rubenstein, MD, MSPH
Professor of Medicine, VA Greater Los Angeles and UCLA
PI, HSR&D Center of Excellence for the Study of Healthcare Provider
Senior Scientist, RAND Corporation
Los Angeles and Santa Monica, CA

John W. Williams Jr., MD, MHS
Professor of Medicine and Psychiatry, Durham VA Medical Center and
Duke University
Director, Duke Evidence-Based Practice Center
Durham, NC

Marjorie Danz, MD
Associate Scientist
RAND Corporation and VA Greater Los Angeles
HSR&D Center of Excellence for the Study of Healthcare Provider
Behavior

Paul Shekelle, MD, PhD
Professor of Medicine, VA Greater Los Angeles and UCLA
Director, Evidence-Based Practice Center RAND Corporation
Los Angeles and Santa Monica, CA

Statistician
Marika Suttorp, MS
RAND Corporation, Santa Monica, CA

Research Assistant
Breanne Johnsen, BA
RAND Corporation, Santa Monica, CA

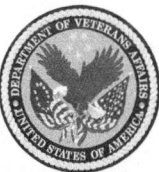

TABLE OF CONTENTS

EVIDENCE SYNTHESIS FOR DETERMINING KEY FEATURES OF EFFECTIVE DEPRESSION INTERVENTIONS

EXECUTIVE SUMMARY

BACKGROUND

Current clinical guidelines for depression address depression treatment for patients detected in primary care (Agency for Health Care Policy and Research 1993; Schulberg, Katon et al. 1998; Agency for Healthcare Policy and Research Depression Guideline Panel 2000); VA/DOD depression guidelines (http://vaww.oqp.med.va.gov); and NICE guidelines (NICE guidelines http://www.nice.org.uk/Guidance/CG23) Research to date indicates that, under usual care conditions, less than half of primary care patients found to have major depression complete minimally adequate medications or psychotherapy (Wells, 2000; Charbonneau, 2003). A variety of organizational changes aimed at improving care for depression in primary care have been tested. Yet evidence-based guidance for healthcare organizations and their primary care practices about which organizational changes are necessary for achieving improved depression outcomes is lacking. The purpose of this review is to establish a basis for organizational guidelines or best practices for achieving improved depression care.

The collaborative care model for depression has been extensively studied, and found to be both effective and cost-effective in prior meta-analysis (Gilbody, Bower et al. 2006; Gilbody, Bower et al. 2006). Collaborative care models are organizational interventions designed to remedy known deficits in current depression care (Hepner, Rowe et al. 2007). These multifaceted models are loosely defined as involving collaboration between providers from different specialties to provide appropriate, timely depression care (Craven, 2002) or as involving two of three types of professionals (a case manager, a primary care clinician, and a mental health specialist) (Gilbody, 2006) working collaboratively within primary care. Thus, while all applications of this model are similar in focusing on supporting effective management of primary care patients detected outside of a mental health specialty setting, the specific features of the model vary from study to study. These variations make it difficult for care settings to know what features of the models tested and found to be effective in randomized trials of collaborative care are essential for achieving the expected effects.

Collaborative care definitions like these have been directed primarily at staffing (e.g., the presence of case manager or mental health specialist). Current theories of chronic illness care, however, postulate that key additional organizational changes are required to achieve consistent, sustainable improvement (Institute of Medicine 2001) (Bodenheimer, 2002). When the multiple facets of collaborative care models are considered, most can be considered specific applications of the general, across-disease chronic illness care model (Wagner, Glasgow et al. 2001). This review focuses on high quality depression care randomized trials that involved at least one change in the organization of care as described in the chronic illness care model (Williams, Gerrity et al. 2007).

Our main research question was whether there are specific design features of collaborative care *interventions* that are consistently associated with greater impact on depression symptoms compared to a usual care control group. We also aimed to explore additional outcomes including patient satisfaction and functioning. In addition, we asked whether there were specific design features of randomized trial evaluations of collaborative care that were associated with consistently greater effects. Secondarily, we aimed to assess whether any patient characteristics, such as comorbidities, were associated with differential collaborative care effects, and the degree to which model effects persisted over time. We investigated these goals based on the following research questions.

1) *Primary Research Question:* **What is the core set of intervention features that characterize collaborative care interventions, and which additional features are most linked to enhanced outcome effects?**

2) *Secondary Research Question:* Are there specific evaluation features among randomized trials of collaborative care that are associated with effect size differences, independently of intervention features?

3) *Secondary Research Question:* To what extent is collaborative care more effective than usual care for decreasing depressive symptoms among patients with comorbid mental health conditions (PTSD, dementia, anxiety, dysthymia, substance abuse) or medical conditions?

METHODS

We used a set of articles identified and preliminarily reviewed as part of an earlier, non-quantitative literature review on depression care models (Williams, Gerrity et al. 2007) to carry out quantitative meta-regression analysis of collaborative care features. Studies were high quality randomized trials of depression collaborative care interventions compared to usual care that incorporated at least two features of the chronic illness care model. At least one of these features had to directly support patients in completing depression treatment. We did not review studies that only sought to change primary care clinician behavior (e.g., using reminders), without an additional patient-directed component, such as care management. We contacted authors extensively to identify, clarify, or verify study variables such as chronic illness care features or patient population characteristics.

We began our analyses by assessing correlations between features. For study outcomes, we evaluated the ***effect size*** across studies for changes in depression symptoms, and ***relative risk*** across studies for changes in rates of resolution of depression. For these analyses we used study effect sizes comparing intervention to usual care arms as the unit of analysis. The effect size analyses treated short (six weeks to four months), medium (five to eight months), and long (nine to twelve months) outcomes separately. We also measured ***intervention impact*** (high, medium, low and little or none) for each study based on reviewer ratings of de-identified sets of study outcomes, including adherence, patient satisfaction, and functioning. We eliminated variables with inadequate distributions for meaningful quantitative analysis, using a rule of thumb of at least three studies per variable category. We carried out univariate and multivariate regression to determine relationships between intervention and evaluation features and effectiveness. .

Finally, we conducted cross-case qualitative analysis (Miles and Huberman 1994) of intervention and evaluation features, including comorbidities, against intervention impact.

RESULTS

Of 1464 articles identified, reviewers deemed 138 as potentially relevant. From this group, we identified 28 high quality randomized controlled trials that met inclusion criteria for collaborative depression care based on the chronic illness care model.

Overall Impact Effectiveness and Impact
Overall, the experimental groups in selected studies showed improvement compared to usual care. Twenty of 28 interventions improved depression outcomes over 3–12 months (an 18.4% median absolute increase in patients with 50% improvement in symptoms; range, 8.3–46%). Because of heterogeneity in outcome time frames and measures across studies, we could not analyze effect sizes for all 28 studies together. Our intervention impact measure enabled us to cross-check our results for all 28 studies as a group. The impact measure was significantly associated with both depression symptom and resolution results as measured using effect size and relative risk.

Regression Results
We found that not all studies could provide suitable information for each effectiveness analysis. 21 of 28 studies were suitable for assessing short-term; 18 for assessing intermediate-term; and 10 for assessing long-term effects on depression symptoms. 18 were suitable for assessing relative risk for depression resolution. We found that studies were too heterogeneous in their assessments of psychiatric comorbidities and demographics to evaluate these variables quantitatively. Too few studies reported on medical comorbidities to evaluate these either qualitatively or quantitatively. We identified some intervention features as too correlated for regression analysis. Initial univariate regression results evaluating the relationship between intervention features and effects on depression symptoms and resolution showed active patient self-management support as the single statistically significant intervention characteristic associated with improved depression symptoms and depression resolution. Other individual collaborative care intervention features among the five we evaluated were not significantly related to outcomes. We found no individual intervention feature associated with longer term effects on depression symptoms. Among evaluation features, enrolling patients for the evaluation through screening was significantly associated with more positive effects on outcomes.

Cross-Case Analysis Results
With between 10 and 21 studies in each regression analysis against study effect size, we did not have the sample size to fully explore potential interactions and associations between intervention features quantitatively. In addition, some variables characterized too large or too small a proportion of the studies to provide adequate variation for valid regression analysis. To understand our initial regression results, we therefore carried out extensive cross-case analyses on our full sample of 28 studies looking at combinations of characteristics versus our impact

measure.

Our cross-case analyses enabled us to evaluate features that occurred together in large proportions of higher impact studies (the 20 studies with high, medium or low impact versus the 8 with little or no impact). We considered features present in 80% or more of the higher impact studies to be core features of effective collaborative care models. Our analyses identified six collaborative care model *intervention* core features. These were:

- Primary care clinicians actively involved in patient management
- Mental health specialists actively involved in patient management
- Care managers assessed patient symptoms at baseline with a standardized scale
- Care managers assessed patient symptoms at follow-up with a standardized scale
- Care managers assessed treatment adherence at follow-up
- Collaborative care intervention included at least 16 weeks of active patient follow-up

We also confirmed our quantitative results regarding patient self-management support. Higher impact studies tended to include active patient self-management support by a care manager or mental health professional, versus passive self-management support such as providing educational brochures.

We found no evaluation design features other than those related to psychiatric comorbidities (excluding bipolar disorder and psychosis) that characterized more than 80% of high impact studies. 77% of high impact studies excluded patients based on substance abuse. Nearly 80% of all 28 studies excluded psychosis and bipolar disorder and nearly all included anxiety. 20% of studies did not mention PTSD; only three of the remaining studies excluded PTSD patients.

CONCLUSIONS

Guidelines for sites intending to implement collaborative care for depression should identify primary care and mental health specialty clinician involvement; care manager assessment of symptoms at baseline and follow-up using a structured instrument; care manager follow-up assessment of treatment adherence; and active follow-up for at least 16 weeks as core features of current evidence-based models. Guidelines should further recommend inclusion of active self-management support, such as elements of patient activation, cognitive behavioral or problem-solving therapy, or motivational techniques, for additional improvement in outcomes. No evidence is available to support using collaborative care for depression with comorbid psychosis or bipolar disorder, and few studies addressed substance abuse. Future research testing collaborative care models for depression should assess effects of medical and psychiatric comorbidities, especially substance abuse.

Evidence Report

INTRODUCTION

Practice improvement to assure appropriate depression care is urgently needed. According to projections from the World Health Organi¬zation, depression will be the second leading cause of disability in the developed world by 2020 (Ormel J 1994; Murray and Lopez 1997). Primary care clinicians (PCCs) care for approximately two thirds of depressed individuals. Rates of optimal quality of care for depression, however, are low (Simon and VonKorff 1995; Hepner, Rowe et al. 2007).

Collaborative care models show promise as guides for achieving appropriate depression care in ordinary primary care practices. These models are organizational interventions that target the structure of primary care practice through changes in elements such as those identified in the Chronic Illness Care Model (Wagner, Austin et al. 2001). A previous rigorously conducted meta-analysis of thirty-seven randomized trials (Gilbody, Bower et al. 2006; Gilbody, Bower et al. 2006) showed the effectiveness of multifaceted interventions based on the collaborative care model (Katon 1995) for improving depression care and outcomes for primary care patients. These studies followed several other literature syntheses on improving care for depression in primary care that drew similar conclusions on the effectiveness of multi-component models (Gilbody, Whitty et al. 2003; Craven and Bland 2006). The success of multi-faceted collaborative care interventions contrasted with prior and subsequent targeted guideline implementation strategies such as screening alone(Goldberg, Steele et al. 1980; Rubenstein, Calkins et al. 1989) , screening plus reminders or management suggestions (Rubenstein, McCoy et al. 1995; Rollman, Hanusa et al. 2002) or education alone(Thompson, Kinmonth et al. 2000).

Not only did collaborative care prove to be effective, it also proved to be cost-effective. A meta-analysis of 11 cost-effectiveness studies on collaborative care showed that the multi-component collaborative care models are within usually accepted ranges of cost-effectiveness, while educational interventions alone are not cost-effective (Gilbody, Bower et al. 2006).

It is important in considering the impact of collaborative care interventions in primary care to recognize that depression of lesser symptom severity or complexity has severe impacts over time if not corrected (Hays, 1995). The effects of depression on job loss (Zhang, Rost et al. 1999; Schoenbaum, Unutzer et al. 2002; Schoenbaum, Sherbourne et al. 2005; Lo Sasso, Rost et al. 2006), social and family relationships, financial decision-making, and other aspects of functioning mean that early in its course, depression can initiate a potentially preventable downward spiral. Thus, effective treatment of the less dramatic presentations of major depression is critical to disability prevention. Yet low complexity patients are less likely to receive appropriate attention under usual care circumstances. Patients with severe depression symptoms and/or psychiatric comorbidities are more likely to be recognized in primary care settings than those with fewer symptoms (Borowsky 2000; Pfaff 2005; Barkow 2004). These complex patients are more likely to be referred to mental health specialists and to comply with the referral as part of usual care (Bartels 2004; Borowsky 2000).

The wealth of evidence on the effectiveness and cost-effectiveness of collaborative care, however, is not matched by a clear understanding of what collaborative care features practices must implement to achieve results similar to the studies. Collaborative care intervention descriptions vary both in terms of what was done and in how intervention features are described. Two meta-analyses of specific intervention features relevant to collaborative care had negative results—i.e., the identified feature was not associated with greater effect sizes. These studies did not directly address collaborative care, but focused on organizational interventions for depression care improvement in primary care. The first was a Cochrane review of the effect of collocation of mental health specialists in primary care (Bower and Sibbald 2000; Mitchell, Del Mar et al. 2002). The second was a study of integration of mental health or substance abuse treatment in primary care (Butler 2008). Thus, to date, there have been no quantitative analyses of features of collaborative care that have been able to clearly identify intervention features associated with effectiveness.

The purpose of this study is to support enhanced implementation of effective collaborative care for depression by identifying key intervention features that are consistently associated with greater impacts on outcomes across the many studies of this model. This will enable the development of practice guidelines, or best practices, that incorporate the best current evidence on the specific organizational features necessary for providing effective care to depressed primary care patients. It will also foster the development of measures of model adherence for use in determining the extent to which collaborative care as implemented matches the key features identified from the literature.

BACKGROUND

Conceptual Approach: Our basic conceptual approach to depression collaborative care was shaped by the chronic illness care model (Fig 1) first described by Wagner et al (Wagner, Austin et al. 2001). We viewed the collaborative care model for depression as a specific case of the chronic illness care model, and identified variables describing study interventions accordingly.

Fig. 1: Chronic Illness Care Model

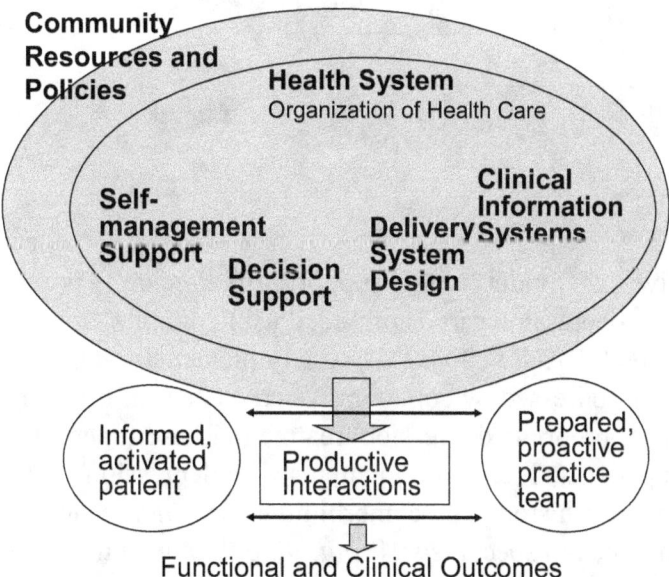

The Chronic Illness Care model postulates types of organizational changes that can support guideline-concordant clinical care. In the case of depression, several specific aspects of depression care highlighted in clinical practice guidelines (Agency for Health Care Policy and Research 1993) are targeted by studies using a Chronic Illness Care type collaborative care approach. These include depression detection (i.e., screening or case finding), assessment (i.e., diagnosis of depression, comorbidities, and contributing factors), proactive follow-up (i.e., contacting patients to support self-management), and mental health specialty input or care for complex patients.

Collaborative Care for Depression: The early studies showing that improved depression outcomes can be achieved by multi-component organizational interventions that support primary care for depression were developed empirically, rather than theoretically. Intervention developers refered to these interventions as depression collaborative care based on their emphasis on linking clinicians and patients in a joint management effort(Katon, Von Korff et al. 1995; Von Korff, Gruman et al. 1997) (Fig. 2). Later developers also emphasized collaboration in terms of the enhancement of links between mental health, primary care, and patients through care management. However, as implemented across a variety of similarly constructed interventions, the term collaborative care has come to incorporate additional features and functions.

Fig. 2: Depression Collaborative Care

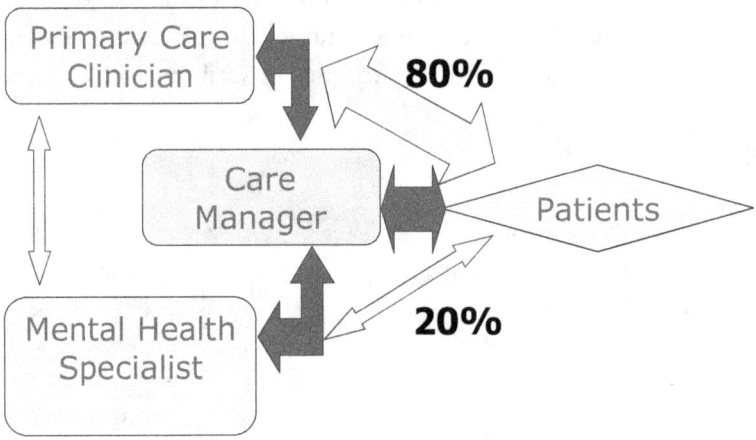

Depression Collaborative Care

In general, collaborative care models aim to support primary care to prevent commonly identified deficits in how depression care is provided using organizational changes, tools, and materials (MacArthur 2003, RAND 2000, IMPACT Implementation Center 2008, Hepner, Rowe et al. 2007). Care deficits addressed by collaborative care occur in fulfilling the **set of functions** necessary for achieving appropriate depression treatment. These functions are:
1) *detecting* depressed patients; 2) *assessing* patients with depression symptoms for depression diagnosis, symptom severity, history, and comorbidities; 3) *triaging* sicker patients to be seen by or followed by mental health specialists; 4) *initiating treatment* that accounts for patient preferences and characteristics; 5) *promoting treatment adherence* through early, active follow-

up; 6) *adjusting treatment* based on patient depression symptom response; and 7) *re-assessing* patient symptoms after treatment to determine need for treatment continuation. All of these activities can be thought of as promoting 8) *patient self-management support.* These functions are difficult to deliver as part of routine primary care. Common barriers are that most patients do not wish to and/or are not able to access mental health specialists; resources for intensive individual mental health specialist care for mildly depressed patients are not available; patient and provider resources for attending primary care as frequently as needed during early treatment are not available; and time and training for primary care clinicians to perform needed symptom and history assessments are not available. Collaborative care models identify organizational resources, as indicated in the chronic illness care model, to overcome these barriers.

Consistent with the chronic illness care model, a major emphasis of collaborative care interventions is *delivery system design.* Typically, these models identify personnel, such as nurses or pharmacists, to fill gaps in usual care for the depression care functions that are most difficult for primary care clinicians to fulfill. These personnel follow designated procedures, usually with identified *decision support,* including provider education. In some cases, *clinical information systems* are engaged to facilitate key functions. *Patient self-management support* is considered important for all patients with chronic illnesses. Depressed patients, however, by virtue of their depressive illness, feel hopeless, helpless, and apathetic—characteristics that promote the low treatment adherence seen in many studies (Katon, von Korff et al. 1992; Lin, Katon et al. 2000). Collaborative care interventions provide patient self management support by promoting pro-active follow-up (i.e., follow-up that is initiated by the provider, rather than the patient); by educating patients; and/or by activating patients through behaviorally-oriented interventions such as problem-solving therapy or cognitive behavioral therapy.

Multifaceted organizational interventions carried out in routine care settings are challenging to synthesize through literature review. These interventions include features adapted to individual organizational settings and resources, preventing uniformity of types of interventions across settings. Echoing findings on collaborative care for depression, we found that multi-faceted organizational interventions targeting Chronic Illness Care Model primary care organizational features such as staffing and delivery system design were more likely to be effective in improving prevention quality than were other types of interventions (Stone, Morton et al. 2002). However, also similarly to prior reviews, we were unable to achieve a high level of specificity about the characteristics of these organizational interventions. Thus, while a strong signal can be detected across broad types of multifaceted interventions, it has been challenging to translate the broad signal into specific guidance for spreading these interventions.

The first set of literature syntheses looked for a signal identifying a general type of depression care improvement intervention with positive effects. These studies identified multi-faceted collaborative care or chronic illness care type interventions as the only general type of intervention to date that had robustly impacted depression outcomes for populations of patients identified as depressed in primary care (Craven and Bland 2002; Gilbody, Whitty et al. 2003). Following this signal, the 2006 Gilbody meta-analysis selected studies based on designation of one or more staff members to support management of depressed patients (care management), and showed overall effectiveness of the 37 selected randomized trials (Gilbody, Bower et al. 2006). A cost effectiveness meta-analysis of a similar set of interventions studies (Gilbody, Bower et al. 2006) showed that these models are relatively inexpensive, may save costs in the long run, and are more cost-effective in terms of benefits to patients than many other commonly-used clinical interventions. All of these literature analyses found that studies varied substantially in the exact configurations of intervention components and features used, as well as in what and how they report on intervention features and outcomes.

In addition to variations in intervention design, studies vary in terms of the patient populations they enroll and in other aspects of their evaluations. For example, some studies include patients screened in as depressed from a primary care population, and referred to collaborative care. Other studies identify patients by asking primary care clinicians or by searching pharmacy data bases for patients recently started on antidepressants. The range of depression symptoms required for inclusion varies from subsyndromal to very severe. Some studies exclude patients with psychiatric comorbidities, while others include them. Most studies exclude the most complex patients. Some studies involve multiple practices, while others focus on only one or two. Some studies involve large practices, often within managed care organizations, while others address small network or private practices. Few studies report in detail on the dynamics of mental health specialty referral or communication (Butler 2008). Overall, little is known about how the variety of possible features affect the chances of impacting patient outcomes.

In this study, we aimed to build on previous reviews using both quantitative and qualitative techniques, combined with extensive queries to authors to obtain unpublished intervention details. We aimed to identify articles that represented organizational change approaches to improving depression care for patients in primary care as emphasized in the chronic illness care model. Based on these, we aimed to describe the set of features that characterize high impact collaborative care interventions as a group. We also aimed to identify a short list of features that, when present, are associated with greater intervention impact. We additionally identified a set of "optional" features that varied across studies but were not associated with differential outcome effects. A short list of such features can assist those implementing collaborative care as a depression quality improvement strategy to choose intervention designs (or change strategies, in quality improvement terminology) with the greatest probability of reproducing the effects of high impact depression care interventions from the literature. Finally, we aimed to add to our current understanding of how to use literature analysis to understand multi-component interventions by using innovative qualitative approaches to overcome some of the methodological limitations of meta-regression for understanding how to implement successful depression collaborative care interventions.

The rationale behind supporting these aspects of depression care delivery is strong, in that depression quality of care is known to be suboptimal in each of these areas, and better performance relative to them is associated with improved outcomes (Hepner, Rowe et al. 2007). To date, collaborative care approaches remain the only identified method for enhancing guideline concordance, and improving outcomes, in primary care. It is thus essential for primary care and mental health specialist managers to know which features of collaborative care research interventions are necessary for achieving effects.

Our study builds directly on a prior literature synthesis recently published by Williams et al. This study aimed at identifying features of collaborative care, but did not carry out quantitative or rigorous qualitative analyses to determine relationships between features and study outcomes.

The data set assembled by this study, however, provides a rigorously identified set of high quality collaborative care articles that follow a chronic illness care model. The authors assembled, in addition, a rich set of over 60 rigorously defined variables, of which 22 related to specific broad intervention or evaluation features. By using this set as a starting point, we aimed to focus this study intensively on understanding the links between features and outcomes.

While previous meta-analyses were aimed primarily at determining whether collaborative care models, loosely defined, were effective, Williams aimed specifically to understand collaborative care features. He and colleagues therefore selected a group of articles that were more homogeneous in design (all randomized trials) and that focused on an organizational intervention aimed at patients (eliminating studies limited to staff level interventions only, such as education or reminders). Selected studies (a) involved primary care patients receiving acute-phase treatment; (b) tested a multicomponent intervention involving at least one patient-directed component; and (c) reported effects on depression severity. Reviewers analyzed the 28 multifaceted organizational interventions meeting these criteria according to intervention features mapped to the Chronic Illness Care Model (Wagner, Austin et al. 2001). Reviewers sought further unpublished details from study authors as needed.

The review found that all selected studies involved care management and required additional resources or staff reassignment to implement. The other most commonly used features among the studies included: patient education and self-management, monitoring of depressive symptoms and treatment adherence, decision support for medication management, a patient registry and mental health supervision of care managers. Additional intervention features were highly variable. Overall, the set of studies selected confirmed prior meta-analysis results, showing significant short-term effects of collaborative care up to 12 months and with three studies showing longer-term effects (up to 57 months). No quantitative analyses relating features to outcomes were performed, however. The study concluded that there was strong evidence supporting the benefits of care management for depression, but only "emerging" evidence on what constituted a successful care management model.

METHODS

Topic Development

The Veterans Health Administration (VHA), along with many other health care organizations and primary care practices, aims to improve care for depression among primary care patients. VHA participated in the President's New Freedom Commission, and developed mental health strategic priorities related to improving mental health care in primary care in 2004 based in part on the Commission's report. Following the strategic plan goals, beginning in 2006, VHA began a series of initiatives focusing on primary care/mental health integration, funded at high levels and culminating in a mandatory Uniform Mental Health Services Package for mental health conditions (VHA Handbook 1160.01). In beginning the improvement process, VHA researchers and policy makers identified the need to understand in more depth which of the features of previously tested multifaceted depression care interventions might be considered optional, and which should be considered required based on their impacts on outcomes. Required features could be incorporated into guidelines or best practices for improvement, and could be targeted for particular attention, tools, and other resources during the implementation of the improvements in new organizations and practices.

Our main research question was whether, based on the literature, there are specific features of rigorously evaluated depression care improvement interventions that characterize effective interventions or are associated with greater intervention impacts. As a secondary research question, we asked whether there were specific design features of the practice settings or of the evaluation designs in these studies that might be associated with consistently greater or smaller effects. We also assessed effects of patient complexity on intervention effectiveness.

METHODOLOGICAL OVERVIEW

In this study, we used the Williams review (Williams, Gerrity et al. 2007) as the basis for further investigation of relationships between intervention features, study designs, and outcomes. We used the 28 selected studies, and the 22 specific variables already abstracted to describe intervention or evaluation features, as the basis for quantitative evaluation. We developed hypotheses about features most likely to affect outcomes, and used existing variables, derived variables based on them, or new variables created for this review to address these hypotheses. We re-abstracted articles and queried authors to complete new variables. All new variables represented independent review and consensus among three investigators (JW, LR, MS). After reviewing quantitative results, we used qualitative cross-case impact analysis (Miles and Huberman 1994) iteratively with quantitative regression analysis to refine our results and develop a short list of key intervention features.

SEARCH STRATEGY

The search strategy used in the Williams review (Williams, Gerrity et al. 2007) is listed below:

DATABASE SEARCHED & TIME PERIOD COVERED:
We searched Medline, HealthSTAR, CINAHL, PsycINFO and a specialized registry of depression trialsfor English-language medical literature published from 1966 to February 2006

LIMITERS:

SEARCH STRATEGY: Search terms included: (a) the MESH terms "depressive disorder" and "depression"; (b) a series of terms validated to identify clinical trials; and (c) a series of MESH terms and text words designed to identify studies using one or more elements of care management (Appendix A). Other sources were references identified from pertinent articles and contacts with experts in the field of depression and health services interventions. Exact search terms are reported in (Williams, Gerrity et al. 2007).
In addition to our PubMed search, we performed reference mining of retrieved articles, references of prior reviews, and solicited articles from experts.

NUMBER OF ITEMS RETRIEVED: 1464

STUDY SELECTION

Of 1464 articles identified, reviewers from the Williams study (Williams, Gerrity et al. 2007) identified 138 as potentially relevant. These were reviewed to identify randomized controlled trials meeting the following selection criteria: (a) samples comprising adult patients with a depressive disorder who were cared for in a primary care setting; (b) interventions needed to augment usual care by incorporating at least one patient-directed element from the CCM (e.g., patient self-management, active follow-up); and (c) studies had to report clinically meaningful outcomes, such as change in depressive symptoms. Interventions directed solely at the clinician (e.g., clinician education or performance feedback) or health care system (e.g., automated clinical reminders) were not included. Twenty-eight of the 136 articles met these criteria.

DATA ABSTRACTION

Our final set of key intervention variables, and their definitions, is listed in Table 1. Some variables are from the original Williams study (Williams, Gerrity et al. 2007). Others are based on either re-derivation or re-abstraction as a part of this study. Table 1 provides the variable labels, names and definitions for the major analytic variables. It also indicates whether the distribution of each variable was adequate for regression analysis (at least 3 studies per variable value) at each time period (short-term, medium-term or long-term). Variables measuring non-white status and comorbidity are listed in Table 7 only.

Variable Definition and Abstraction in the Williams Study: In the Williams study (Williams, Gerrity et al. 2007) pairs of independent reviewers (SKD, AJD, JWW, JD, TH, BNG) abstracted the 28 articles to identify features of the chronic illness care model (Wagner, Austin et al. 2001; Bodenheimer, Wagner et al. 2002; Bodenheimer, Wagner et al. 2002); study clinician and patient characteristics; 3) components of the intervention (decision support, self-management support, delivery system redesign including care management and enhanced mental health involvement, and clinical information systems), and support for implementing the intervention; 4) care management functions and process, and 5) outcomes. When key information was missing or unclear, investigators contacted the primary author for clarification; 22 of 24 authors contacted responded to our request. Two investigators (MSG, JWW) reviewed areas of disagreement. Final classification was based on the consensus of all investigators.

Data abstraction included study design features, including inclusion and exclusion criteria, and proportion of minorities in the study. The study also focused substantially on care management, defined as any systematic or structured management of patient care by a designated provider, and on patient outcomes. Specific abstracted features on care management included coordination and communication among treating health care providers, patient education, monitoring symptoms and adherence to treatment plans, self-management support, or psychological treatments (Katon, Von Korff et al. 2001; Oxman, Dietrich et al. 2002). Outcomes abstracted included the proportion of subjects who had a least a 50% decrease in depressive symptomatology or remission in symptoms based on a validated questionnaire, the mean change in depressive symptoms, and antidepressant adherence. Extensive variable tables are included in the Williams publication.

Study Intervention and Evaluation Variable Definition and Abstraction (Current Study): We reviewed, re-abstracted or re-defined variables from the Williams study related to four categories relevant to our research questions. The first category focused on study intervention features and patient characteristics. The second category focused on intervention features. The third category focused on measures of study impact, including depression symptoms, patient adherence to treatment, satisfaction, and global improvement or functioning. The fourth category focused on study design characteristics, including proportion of patients who were non-white, and inclusion and exclusion criteria.

We then derived ten new variables. Five of the new variables required re-abstraction of the article set, while the other five were new combinations of previous variable values. Variables we re-derived and/or re-reviewed included those related to 1) care management (defined as any systematic or structured management of patient care that included coordination and communication among treating health care providers); 2) patient education; 3) self-manage¬ment support or psychological treatments; 4) monitoring of symptoms; 5) monitoring of adherence to treatment plans, and 6) impact.

We contacted authors for additional information as needed. Overall, between the original data collection and our final data collection effort, we attempted to contact all but two of the authors, and succeeded in getting a responses from all but one of those we attempted (26/28). We got information from each of these authors between one and four times (mean 2.1). Only one of the authors contacted was unable to supply the information we needed. In both the original and final data collection efforts, two investigators independently abstracted the articles and reviewed any area of disagreement. Final variable values in the original data set were based on the consensus of all investigators on that article, and in our additional data collection were based on consensus of two authors (Williams and Rubenstein). For final analyses, a third author (MS) reviewed variables we identified as significant.

Study Outcome Variable Definitions and Abstraction: We used effect sizes for depression symptom change and relative risk of depression resolution as our main outcome measures. Our statistician for this study (MS) independently abstracted the data needed to calculate both effect sizes for the continuous outcomes and risk ratios for the dichotomous outcomes.

Our symptom outcome variables identified all reported *effect sizes* in *short* (six weeks to four months), *medium* (five to eight months), and *long* (nine to twelve months) time strata after baseline. We developed one set of outcome variables with values at these time periods based on continuous symptom measures, and another set based on dichotomous outcomes. Examples of continuous outcomes include results based on depression scales such as the Beck Depression Inventory, Hamilton Depression Rating Scale, or Hopkins Symptoms Checklist-20). Examples of dichotomous outcomes include assessments of the percent of patients recovered or below a specified symptom threshold by the end of the study.

After initial hypothesis testing, we developed and validated a newly-developed *impact scale* for subsequent qualitative and quantitative analyses. Because studies used different symptom measures and different follow-up time periods, each outcome variable based on effect size included only a portion of the articles in the set. To create an outcome measure applicable to all articles in the set, we developed an impact rating for each article.

To derive the impact measure, we randomly ordered the 28 studies on an Excel spreadsheet and listed only each study's set of outcomes, without any other identifiers. We listed all of the measured outcomes for each study that fell into one of four conceptual domains. These were depression symptom outcomes, process of care outcomes (usually adherence to antidepressants), patient satisfaction, and quality of life or functioning (see table below). For each outcome we listed whatever statistics the authors reported. Two authors (LR and JW) then independently reviewed and rated the outcomes on the scrambled Excel spreadsheet, independently of any article identifiers. One investigator (JW) rechecked using outcomes from Table 4, Williams (Williams 2007). Considerations for assigning impact level included consistency of results across domains, size and significance of the effects, and persistence of results over time. The rating process graded impacts on a four-point scale as robust (high), medium, low, and none or negative. Interater reliability for impact judgments was high, with agreement on 86% (24/28) of ratings. Final impact ratings reflected consensus on the four studies rated differently. The example table below shows four actual example studies with their impact ratings.

EXAMPLE TABLE FOR HOW IMPACT RATINGS WERE CARRIED OUT

Example Studies	Treatment Adherence (short-term)	Treatment Adherence (medium term)	Depression Symptoms (short term)	Depression Symptoms (medium or long term)	Satisfaction	Global or Functional Impact	Impact Rating By LR, JW
Information recorded for each study, as available. Usual care group noted first vs. intervention group	E.g., odds ratios, significance, what was measured, time measured	E.g., odds ratios, significance, what was measured, time measured	E.g., odds ratios, change scores, significance, patients with 50% symptom decrease, type of measure,	E.g., odds ratios, change scores, significance; patients with 50% symptom decrease; type of measure	E.g., odds ratios, percent satisfied, significance, time measured	E.g., odds ratios, significance, what was measured	Robust, Moderate, Weak, Little or No Impact
#1	---	----	-3.9 vs -5.6, p= .02, Ham-D change, 3 mos.	-4.0, vs -7.3 p<.001, Ham-D change, 6 mos. 33% vs, 53% p<.001, Ham-D 50% improvement, at 12 mos.	----	P < .05 on the SF 20 at 12 mos., exact score not given	Robust
#2	957 vs 867, NS, Mean milligrams antidepressant dispensed at 6 wks	2267i vs. 2111, NS, Mean milligrams antidepressant dispensed at 6 mos	33% vs 38%, p=.01, Ham-D 50% improvement, at 6 weeks 33% vs 38%, NS, Beck 50% improvement, at 6 wks.	38% vs. 57%, p=.003, Ham-D 50% improvement at 6 mos. 37% vs. 48%, p = .05, Beck 50% improvement at 6 wks.	3.94 vs. 4.20, p=.001, 11 item unpublished scale, at 6 mos.	44.6 vs. 47.3, p = .10, SF-12 MCS score at 6 mos.	Moderate
#3	--	42% vs 64%., p<.001, prescribed >90 days AD	1.5 vs. 1.58, NS, SCL-20, at six months	1.63 vs. 1.62 NS, SCL-20, at six months	---	31.7 vs. 31.1, NS, PCS from SF36V	Weak
#4	No significant difference at 3 mos. (no numeric data provided)	30% versus 49% adherent to anti-depressants, p ≤.05, at six months excluding 3 dropouts, NS for intent to treat	21% vs. 21% 50% improvement, NS, BDI, 3 mos.	---	---	----	Weak

STUDY QUALITY ASSESSMENT

Determination of study quality was based on the Williams study. The quality measure took account of the process of randomization and allocation concealment, fidelity to the planned intervention without significant co-intervention, follow-up rates and analytic methods, using an intent-to-treat approach and blinded outcome assessments. Based on these criteria, risk of bias was rated as a low (all elements met), moderate (≥ 1 element partially met), or high (≥ 1 element not met) (Higgins and Green). There were no disagreements about quality assessments.

DATA SYNTHESIS AND ANALYSIS

Correlations: Prior to carrying out regression analysis, we evaluated correlations between intervention and evaluation design features. Since intervention and evaluation features were categorical, we evaluated the correlations between variables using cross tabulations and the chi-square statistic.

Effect Size Calculations for Continuous Outcomes: In order to compare estimates across studies that report different depression scales, the effect size was selected as the unit of analysis. An effect size was calculated if the follow-up mean, standard deviation, and sample size for both the intervention group and usual care group were reported or could be calculated. For trials that reported a mean outcome but no standard deviation, the standard deviation was estimated by taking the mean standard deviation weighted by the sample size across all other trials that reported standard deviations for that outcome (Furukawa, 2006).

Only one comparison per study within each time strata was calculated. For studies that included more than one intervention group, the group that was most similar to the complete collaborative care model was included. In addition, only one outcome per study was used. If a study reported more than one depression scale, then the measure that was clinically homogeneous to the scales reported in the other included studies was selected. Effect sizes were calculated by dividing the difference of follow-up means of the intervention and control group by the pooled follow-up standard deviations of the two groups (Sutton AJ, 2000). Ninety-five percent confidence intervals were calculated for each effect size. A negative effect size indicates that the intervention group did better at follow-up than the control group. Negative effect sizes indicate benefit because when the intervention group is doing better than the control group, depression symptoms are reduced. Thus, for example, for each independent variable, the largest negative effect size shows the group with the greatest effect.

Risk Ratio Calculations for Dichotomous Outcomes: We estimated a risk ratio to assess effect for dichotomous variables. For the risk ratio analysis, we used the longest follow-up interval reported. Risk ratios and their ninety-five percent confidence intervals were estimated for studies that reported the percent of people who improved since baseline in each study. A risk ratio greater than one indicates that the intervention group had a higher rate of improvement than the usual care group did. For example, a risk ratio of 1.50 signifies that 50% more people improved in the intervention group than in the usual care group. All analyses were conducted in Stata version 10.0.

Quantitative analysis focused on assessing key independent variables related to evaluation or implementation design against depression symptom outcomes as the dependent variable. Correlations between the independent variables were assessed. A stratified meta-regression was conducted separately for each independent variable with the effect size as the outcome (Sutton AJ, 2000). Stratification was based on follow-up time. A study could contribute to more than one stratum. Bivariate meta-regressions using the same independent variables as above were also conducted using the risk ratio as the outcome. Estimates were obtained from the meta-regessions for each level of the independent variable. In most cases, the independent variables had two levels (e.g. did the study have the component or not). A z-test was used from the meta-regression to test if the difference in effect sizes or risk ratios was significant between component groups. Differences with p-values less than 0.05 were denoted (Stata, 2006).

In this study, we found variations in which outcomes were used, ranging from a variety of depression symptom indices, health-related quality of life, patient satisfaction, and process of care for depression. We also found variations in when outcomes were measured. We used a conservative analytic approach such that we focused on depression symptom outcomes only. We also focused on time frames separately, rather than combining results across time frames.

QUALITATIVE ANALYSIS

We carried out qualitative cross-case analysis using methods based on Miles and Huberman (Miles and Huberman 1994). We used this approach to overcome limitations to meta-regression in our article sample—primarily the inability to include all 28 selected articles in a single meta-regression analysis. In traditional meta-analysis, the study intervention is treated as the same across all studies. The major challenges posed during this kind of analysis derive from variations in how outcomes are reported (e.g. by time period, or specific measure); these variations may limit the number of studies included in a given analysis. However, since each study is included as a whole, power for detecting overall effects with an article sample size like ours is generally adequate. Meta-regression, however, makes comparisons within the overall group of studies and is thus more analytically demanding. In addition, valid meta-regression using multiple features or control variables simultaneously would require more studies than were available to us. Since no single quantitative outcome analysis in this study included all reviewed studies, we wanted to confirm qualitatively that our quantitative results were insensitive to inclusion of all studies in the same outcome analysis. We also wanted to be able to assess intervention features that characterized too many studies in the sample to be tested quantitatively (see Table 1). Cross-case analysis afforded us the ability to achieve these goals.

To carry out the analyses, we ranked studies by impact level based on our overall impact measure (see above). We focused primarily on the intervention features that had inadequate distributions either at all time periods or at medium-term and long-term due to being present in too many studies in the sample (see Table 1). These intervention characteristics could not be adequately tested quantitatively. We also developed four main scenarios based on our hypotheses for types of interventions or design features and their relationships to impact. We then created a series of tables around these scenarios as antecedent matrices related to our conceptual model of collaborative care and our hypotheses about effects of study design features. We looked for patterns, and verified scenarios for similar and contrasting outcomes.

PEER REVIEW

This report was reviewed by our technical experts. Their comments were taken into consideration in our revision. Service as a technical expert does not imply endorsement of the report's findings. A table of peer review comments received and the changes we made to the report is presented in Appendix B.

RESULTS

LITERATURE FLOW

Of 138 studies reviewed, 29 met all inclusion criteria (Fig. 1). One of these was excluded because the intervention targeted relapse prevention for patients in remission from a depressive episode. Twenty-eight studies were reviewed for further analysis. Reviewers also consulted fifty-six articles that were companion papers for included studies and described methods, long-term outcomes, subgroup analyses, cost data and other outcomes.

Among the 28 selected studies, overall study quality was high (Table 2 and Appendix A). Risk of bias was low in 18/28 studies (64%); moderate in 6/28(22%); and high in 4/28 (14%). Outcomes were assessed blind to treatment assignment in 23 studies, and intent-to-treat analyses were used in 21 studies. Fifteen of the 28 studies (54%) involved managed care practices, including five in Veterans Affairs facilities. Most were carried out in the United States.

STUDIES INCLUDED IN EFFECT SIZE OR RELATIVE RISK ANALYSES

Twenty-five of the 28 studies included usable continuous depression symptom measures for analysis, while three studies did not. Two of the excluded studies did not report a follow-up mean, and one did not report the sample size by group. Among the 25 studies in the continuous measure analysis, 21 included effect sizes based on short-term follow-up. Eighteen studies contributed intermediate-term effect sizes. Ten studies contributed long-term effect sizes. Eighteen studies reported a dichotomous improvement outcome and were included in the risk ratio analysis.

Four studies had two intervention arms and reported results for each arm separately. For Katon (1995) and Katon (1996) the major depression groups were used while the minor depression groups were excluded. Simon (2004) reported two intervention groups. Both had telephone care management. One group had the addition of telephone psychotherapy which was the intervention group we selected to compare against the usual care group. Simon (2000) had feedback only and care management – we selected the care management group to compare to the usual care group. For Wells (2000), the enhanced medication arm was used.

We found that not all studies could provide suitable information for each effectiveness analysis. We found that studies were too heterogeneous in their assessments of comorbidities and demographics to evaluate any of these variables quantitatively. We were, however, able to evaluate studies with a higher proportion (over 25%) minorities. 6 studies did not report minority status.

CORRELATIONS BETWEEN FEATURES
When we evaluated correlations between the intervention and evaluation features used in our final analyses, we found that enrolling patients through primary care clinician referral of patients or by identification of patients on antidepressants (versus by screening) is significantly correlated

with use of patient level randomization (p = .03). Enrolling patients referred by primary care clinicians on antidepressants or willing to take them is correlated with study inclusion of fewer practice groups.(p = .01). Having mental health specialists involved in patient management was also correlated with inclusion of fewer practice groups (p = .03).

Looking just at collaborative care model intervention features, we found that studies in which medications were adjusted by primary care clinicians with expert guidance were significantly more likely to include care managers who were nurses, versus other types of professionals; were more likely to include at least 16 weeks of follow-up (p = .04); used more intensive (robust) interventions (p = .001); and followed an overall classic collaborative care intervention model (p = .04). Classic collaborative care interventions were correlated with having a dedicated care manager who used standardized depression symptom scales for follow-up (p = .03). Including active self-management was correlated with having a dedicated depression care manager who assessed depression symptoms with a structured instrument at baseline and at one or more follow-up visits, and who also assessed treatment adherence (p = .02).

No other correlations (associations) between study variables shown in Table 1 were significant at p <.05.

OVERALL EFFECTIVENESS

Overall, the experimental groups in selected studies showed improvement. The overall effect size by follow-up time was: short-term, -0.28 (-0.38, -0.19); intermediate term, -0.25 (-0.37, -0.14); and long-term, -0.19 (-0.36, -0.02). Twenty of 28 interventions improved depression outcomes over 3–12 months (an 18.4% median absolute increase in the proportion of patients with 50% improvement in symptoms; range, 8.3–46%).

STUDY EVALUATION DESIGN FEATURES VS. EFFECTIVENESS

Study designs varied on several major features. Subjects were recruited using four strategies: screening (n =11), clinician referral (n =9), administrative or pharmacy databases (n =3), a combination of these strategies (n =3) or direct contact by a pharmacist when an antidepressant prescription was filled (n =2). The unit of randomization varied across studies: 18 randomized patients, 3 randomized providers and 7 randomized practices.

Table 3 shows the relationship between four evaluation design features and depression symptoms and resolution, using univariate regression. In the table, the group with the higher negative effect size shows greater reduction in depression symptoms, and the group with the higher relative risk shows a better chance of depression resolution. Because nearly all studies had some effect, effect sizes both with and without the target feature are negative (showing an effect on depression symptoms), and nearly all relative risks are greater than one (showing greater resolution of depression). We report results on short-term, medium-term, and long-term outcomes. Our results show that studies in which patients were referred to care management through screening, rather than by primary care clinicians or administrative medication records, had a significantly higher relative risk of depression resolution. No other among the four design features we investigated was significantly linked to outcomes.

Table 3 also shows that studies with greater than 25% minorities tended to show greater effects, although this difference did not reach statistical significance. Six studies did not record minority status.

ASSOCIATIONS BETWEEN INTERVENTION FEATURES AND OUTCOME EFFECT SIZES

Table 4a shows the relationship between nine variables reflecting collaborative care model intervention features and depression symptoms and resolution. In the table, the group with the higher negative effect size shows greater reduction in depression symptoms, and the group with the higher relative risk shows a better chance of depression resolution. We report results on short-term, medium-term, and long-term outcomes. Initial univariate regression results evaluating the first five individual features listed in the table (structured care manager assessment, active self-management support, care manager triage to mental health, adjustment of antidepressants by primary care clinicians, and care managers who were predominantly nurses) showed active patient self-management support as the single statistically significant intervention characteristic associated with improved depression symptoms and depression resolution.

We then derived additional variables shown in Table 4b. This table shows that studies with nurse or PhD pharmacist care management, patient education, and at least sixteen weeks of care manager follow-up (classic collaborative care model with long-term follow-up, see variables Table 1) are associated with significantly improved long-term effects on depression symptoms. Having at least 16 weeks of care manager follow-up alone was not well-distributed as a variable, but appeared to be associated with a significantly greater reduction in depression symptoms at short-term and medium-term time points.

IMPACT MEASURE

We designed our study impact measure to distinguish between high, medium or low impact by the study intervention by qualitatively taking into account all key outcome variables comparing intervention to usual care and all measurement time periods. We therefore expected it to be associated with, but not identical to, our quantitative study effect size measures of depression symptom reductions. Though the impact measure was based on expert rating, it was significantly associated with quantitative depression symptom effect size results at each time point (Table 5). Based on quantitative depression symptom reduction effects, the impact measure statistically distinguished studies designated as showing high, medium, or low impact from those designated as showing little or no impact. The impact measure was also associated with significantly greater relative risk of depression resolution. However, unlike the effect size measures we used for our primary study outcome tests, and as discussed in the Methods section above, the impact measure could be applied to all 28 studies. This afforded us additional opportunities to evaluate our results, and test their sensitivity to inclusion of all studies together.

QUALITATIVE ANALYSIS OF INTERVENTION FEATURES VERSUS OUTCOME IMPACTS

To understand our initial regression results, we carried out extensive cross-case analyses looking at combinations of characteristics versus our impact measure, based on a priori study questions as indicated in Methods above. Table 6 shows cross-case analysis of our key collaborative care model intervention features. The cross-case analyses enabled us to look closely at features that occurred together in large proportions of higher impact studies (the 20 studies with high, medium or low impact versus the 8 with little or no impact). We considered features present in 80% or more of the higher impact studies to be core features of effective collaborative care models. Our analyses identified six collaborative care model intervention core features. These were:

- Primary care clinicians actively involved in patient management
- Mental health specialists actively involved in patient management
- Care managers assessed patient symptoms at baseline with a standardized scale
- Care managers assessed patient symptoms at follow-up with a standardized scale
- Care managers assessed treatment adherence at follow-up
- Collaborative care intervention included at least 16 weeks of active patient follow-up

As shown in Table 6 and, in greater detail, in Table 9, active patient self-management support strongly characterized the high and medium impact studies, and became less prevalent in the low and little or no impact groups. Only one high impact study and only two medium impact studies did not undertake active self-management support. The one high impact study without active patient self-management (Katzelnick, Simon et al. 2000) used a previously tested and validated educational tool.

As indicated in Table 6, there were five VA studies in the sample, and one additional study with a VA site. Among the studies conducted in Veterans Affairs facilities, those that supported active patient self-management (Oslin, Sayers, Ross, et al., 2003; Fortney, Pyne, Edlund, et al., 2006) had the higher impact scores. One study (Swindle) that had low impact used mental health clinical nurse specialists as care managers and did not include structured assessment. A second low impact VA study (Dobscha) did not include at least twelve weeks of follow-up.

Table 9 shows the details of the self-management support interventions used in these studies. While all included studies incorporated at least one chronic illness care element directed toward patients, this element might be, for example, care manager assessment without patient education and behavioral activation. We looked for self-management support approaches that featured behavioral activation or interactive problem-solving approaches, usually in addition to standard patient education using written material or videotapes. We counted CBT provided by mental health specialists as therapy rather than self-management support.

In addition to core features, we used qualitative analyses to identify features that varied across high impact studies, and could thus be considered options. The main feature that emerged as an option was telephone versus in person care management.

QUALITATIVE ANALYSIS OF EVALUATION DESIGN FEATURES, IN-CLUDING PATIENT COMORBIDITY, VERSUS OUTCOME IMPACTS

Table 8 shows qualitative results for evaluation design features. We found no evaluation design features other than those related to comorbidities that characterized more than 80% of high impact studies. In general, studies conducted in Veterans Affairs facilities were medium-sized, randomized at the provider or practice level, and eligible patients were referred through screening.

Table 7 shows results for comorbidities and demographics versus impact. More than 80% of studies excluded patients with bipolar disorder and psychosis. No study excluded anxiety. Six studies (21%) did not mention PTSD, and only 14% of the remaining 22 studies excluded patients based on it. Most studies (18 of the 28) excluded patients with substance abuse. Six studies (21%) did not report on the proportion of minorities enrolled.

In evaluating the relationship between evaluation design features and outcomes, we found no consistent effects qualitatively for the following design variables: number of practices in the study, patients per practice, whether patients were screened by the study and referred or were referred by their clinicians, or whether randomization was at the patient or cluster level.

LIMITATIONS

The results of this review are limited by several important factors. First, the analyses conducted in this paper were not designed to address causality. Even the quantitative analyses must be considered descriptive, and the qualitative analyses are hypothesis-generating. The number of categories of analytic variables tested and the possibility of misclassification of variables across reviewers have the potential to bias our results. With only 28 articles, quantitative analyses are of necessity limited. Nevertheless, within the framework of a set of complex interventions that we already know have robust effects on depression outcomes, but that vary in basic components, our analyses have substantial strengths. Strengths of our analyses include our extensive querying of authors regarding intervention and evaluation features; our systematic approach to analysis; our rigorous variable definitions and validation through independent review and consensus; and our triangulation, or sensitivity testing, of conclusions across methodologies.

Our qualitative approach is hypothesis generating. Our impact score is subjective, although rigorously derived and associated with effect sizes at each time frame. However, the only quantitative approach to defining an outcome across all 28 studies would have been to combine effects across heterogeneous time frames and measurement methods, an approach that may have resulted in greater bias than the method we chose. Future studies could assess the tradeoffs between these approaches. Our analysis is based on iterative review of data by investigators, and thus subject to bias. Our use of rigorous cross-case methods mitigates, but does not eliminate this possibility. The transparent presentation of our analyses to readers in tabular form, however, should assist readers in making independent assessments of our conclusions.

The studies upon which we based our analyses also have limitations. The studies themselves have selection biases. Even studies that use screening to identify patients exclude some categories of patients and recruit only a portion of those eligible due to refusal. We therefore cannot be certain how well these studies generalize to use of the collaborative care model in usual practice settings. Most interventions in these studies were imple¬mented through large health care organizations, limiting the generalizability of the results to organizations with sufficient structure, commitment and resources to imple¬ment interventions requiring changes in systems of care. Moreover, practices in fee-for-service environments that do not reimburse for care management services have fewer incentives for implementing these interventions. In addition, there may be contextual variables not measured in the studies that influence outcomes. For example, even within managed care organiza¬tions, Rubenstein et al. (Rubenstein, Parker et al. 2002; Rubenstein, Meredith et al. 2006) found that expert leadership and support from local practice management and mental health specialists influenced the development of successful programs. In addition, study comparisons were to usual care. Usual care, however, is heterogeneous across settings and providers, For example, some usual care settings may have ample mental health specialty access, while some have little.

In terms of the interventions studied, we could not test the independence of many of the features in association with outcomes because the features were not distributed evenly among studies. Some features also tended to occur with other features. We extensively tested combinations of features both in quantitative analysis (e.g., the classic collaborative care model) and in qualitative analysis, where features could be viewed as present or absent across studies.

Our study is limited in terms of shedding light on the chronic illness care model as applied to conditions other than depression. Depression has unique features that might make it more necessary to expend resources on, for example, care management. Depressed patients tend to be apathetic, poor consumers who benefit from proactive care. They are often not detected without screening. Screening requires psychological testing, rather than a blood test, and follow-up of positive screens requires either a full mental health specialist interview or psychological assessments using standardized tests that take in the neighborhood of 40 minutes to complete. Assessment is difficult to complete in an average 20 minute primary care visit. Assessment can additionally uncover serious urgent or emergent conditions such as suicidal threats, requiring additional time to handle appropriately. Furthermore, adherence to treatment is likely to be a more prevalent problem among depressed patients than among other chronically ill patients. Follow-up care requires frequent contact, but not full in-person visits—the interview, not the physical examination or laboratory testing, provides most of the necessary information. Finally, mental health specialists may be more organizationally or geographically separate from primary care than are other specialists. The unique characteristics of depression may thus help explain why there is substantially more evidence for cost-effectiveness of depression collaborative care than for other care management-based interventions. Future research will clarify the transportability of conclusions on depression collaborative care to other chronic conditions.

The studies on collaborative care for depression were also severely limited in terms of addressing medical or psychiatric comorbidities. No evidence is available from these studies on collaborative care for bipolar disorder or psychosis, because these patients were nearly universally excluded. Patients with subthreshold depression were also usually excluded, although one of the studies later found evidence of positive effects among these patients (Wells 2005). Only a few studies included patients with substance abuse. Among the studies that included a broader group of patients, intervention protocols most likely specified referring patients with severe psychiatric comorbidities for mental health specialty care (e.g., RAND 2000). Thus, no conclusions can be drawn from this review on collaborative care for primary care patients with medical or psychiatric comorbidities.

This study identified only 28 studies out of 1464 that met full inclusion criteria, and less than half of these were published in the last five years. Previous collaborative care literature syntheses have netted 30 to 40 includes, but have included more heterogeneous groups of interventions and evaluations. New methods for achieving the necessary improvements in depression care may well be identified in future reviews.

CONCLUSIONS

While collaborative care models for depression vary, careful analysis of model features shows that a core set of characteristics is linked to better results. This set is robust across qualitative and quantitative analyses, and does not seem to be biased by links to particular evaluation design features (e.g., the design feature of randomization at the patient level is distributed across all levels of care model impact). In addition to the core variables, active patient self management support appears to characterize the set of very high impact studies. These finding are sufficiently strong to support recommendations to sites intending to implement collaborative care for depression.

Guidelines for sites intending to implement collaborative care for depression should identify primary care and mental health specialty clinician involvement; care manager assessment of symptoms at baseline and follow-up using a structured instrument; care manager follow-up assessment of treatment adherence; and active follow-up for at least 16 weeks as core features of current evidence-based models. Guidelines should further recommend inclusion of active self-management support, such as elements of patient activation, cognitive behavioral or problem-solving therapy, or motivational techniques, for additional improvement in outcomes.

Figure 1. Article Flow

Relevant studies (n = 138)

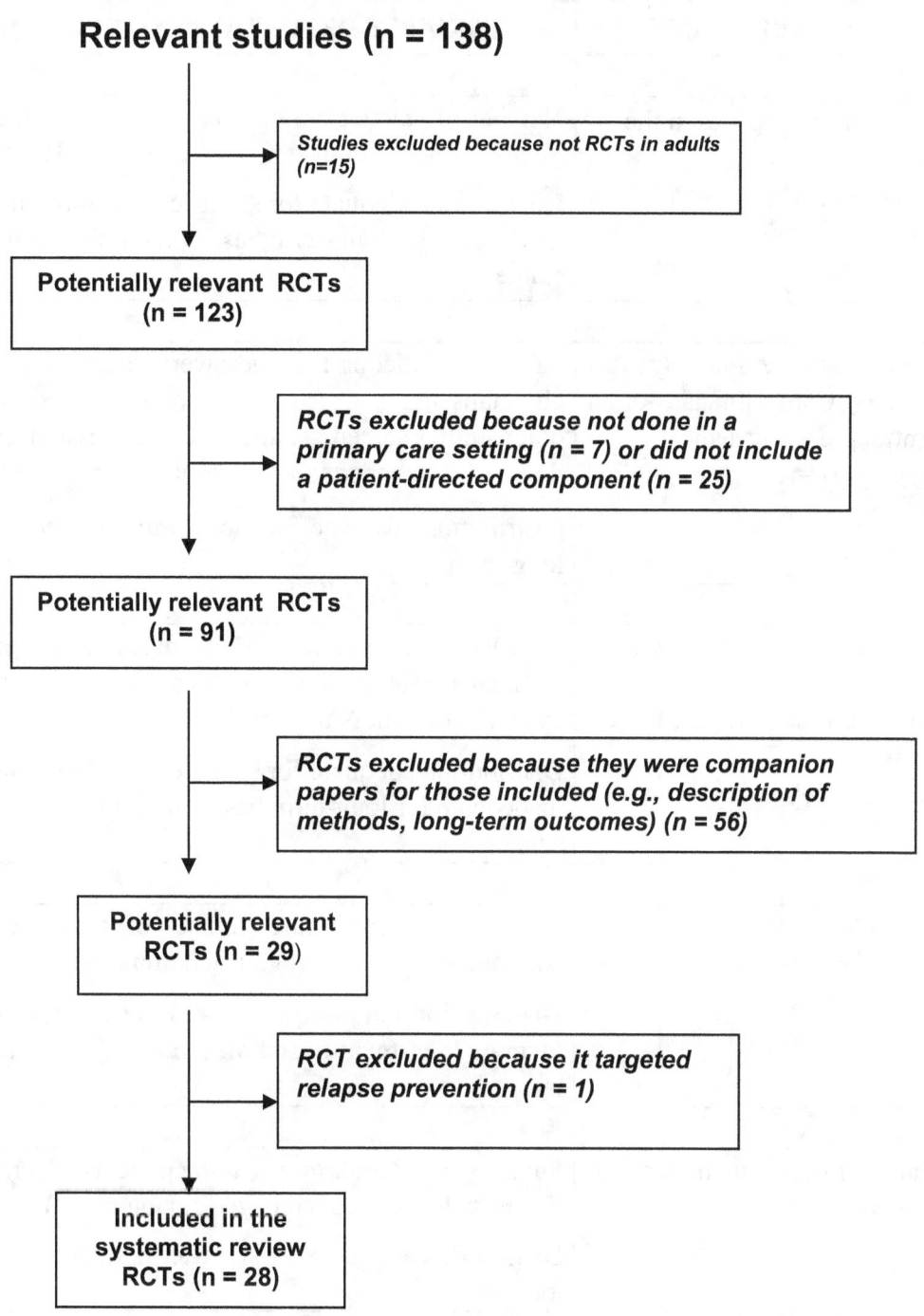

Fig. 1. Flow diagram of the search and selection processes for trials included in the systematic review.

Table 1: Variables Characterizing the Study Intervention and Design

VARIABLE NAME	VARIABLE DEFINITION AND DISTRIBUTION†
Number of Practices in the Study *(practice group = small, medium, or large)*	Number of practices in the study. There are three levels: Small (1-2); Medium = (3-10); Large = (>10). (categorical) Distribution adequate for short-term and intermediate-term. Inadequate for long-term based on too few "small" category studies.
Referred to the Study by Primary Care Clinicians or on Antidepressant Medications *(type_ref1=yes)*	Patients enrolled in the study were referred by primary care clinicians and/or were on antidepressant medications. All other studies screened patients for depression, and included those who screened in as probably depressed. (dichotomous) Distribution adequate for short-term, intermediate-term and long-term.
Referred to the Study by Primary Care Clinicians and on Antidepressant Medications or Willing to Take Them. *(type_ref2=yes)*	Patients enrolled in the study were referred by primary care clinicians and were on antidepressant medications or indicated a willingness to start them. Distribution adequate for short-term and intermediate-term; inadequate for long-term based on too few "yes" category studies.
Study Set in Primary Care Clinician Offices *(type_set=yes)*	Study set in primary care clinician offices rather than in a community-based setting. (dichotomous) **Distribution not adequate for short-term, intermediate-term or long-term based on too few "no" category studies.**
Patient Level Randomization *(rand1=yes)*	Subjects were randomized at the patient level rather than at the provider or practice level (dichotomous) Distribution adequate for short-term, intermediate-term and long-term.

VARIABLE NAME	VARIABLE DEFINITION AND DISTRIBUTION†
Structured Care Manager Assessment of Depression Symptoms (Baseline and Follow-up) and Treatment Adherence (CMAssess= yes)*	Depression Care Manager (DCM) assesses depression symptoms with a structured instrument at baseline and at one or more follow-up visits; and also assesses treatment adherence (dichotomous) Distribution adequate for short-term and intermediate-term but not for long-term, based on too few "no" category studies.
Active Self-Management Support (self_manage = yes))	Facilitates active self-management (goal-setting and/or patient activation), provides patient education, and encourages adherence to plan and tracking of progress (dichotomous) Distribution adequate for short-term, intermediate-term and long-term.
Care Manager Triage to Mental Health (MH_spec=yes)	DCM guided patients to mental health specialty instead of primary care based on preferences, symptoms, co-morbidities, or other clinical judgment (dichotomous) Distribution adequate for short-term, intermediate-term and long-term.
Primary Care Clinician Adjusts Antidepressants (MedAdjR=yes)	Primary care clinician adjusted antidepressant medications with review and input as needed from a mental health specialist or other depression medication expert (dichotomous) Distribution adequate for short-term and intermediate-term, but not for long-term, based on too few "no" category studies.
Care Managers are Medical Nurses (CMMedNurse=yes)	Care managers were predominantly medical nurses rather than psychiatric nurses, other mental health professionals, pharmacists, or health educators (dichotomous) Distribution adequate for short-term, intermediate-term and long-term.

VARIABLE NAME	VARIABLE DEFINITION AND DISTRIBUTION†
Intensity of Intervention Assessment and Follow-Up *(robustness=high, medium, or low)*	Intensity is defined by three features: (1) DCM structured assessment of depression symptoms (baseline and follow-up) and treatment adherence, (2) adequate number (mean of >3) of DCM contacts, and (3) antidepressant adjustment by the primary care clinician with expert guidance. The three levels of intensity are based on having one, two, or three features (categorical) Distribution adequate for short-term, but not for intermediate-term or long-term based on too few "medium" category studies.
Classic Collaborative Care Intervention With Long Follow-up *(type_int1= yes)*	Has care management by an RN or doctoral level pharmacist, primary care clinician collaboration with mental health specialty, patient education, and follow-up for at least 16 weeks (either by telephone or in person) (dichotomous) Distribution adequate for short-term, intermediate-term and long-term.
Active Patient Follow-up for At Least 16 Weeks *(_16_weeks = yes)*	Intervention included at least 16 weeks of active patient follow-up (dichotomous) **Distribution adequate for short-term, but not for intermediate-term or long-term based on too few "no" category studies.**
Overall Intervention Impact *(impact = high (1), medium (2), low (3), little or no (4))*	Independent judgment regarding how certain and how large the impact of the intervention was by two reviewers blinded to study methods or results (viewing extracted study outcomes only). Raters identified four levels of impact (high, medium, low, and little or no impact). Judgments were based on effect size/significance of intervention impact on depression symptoms, process of care, patient satisfaction, and overall quality of life, considering all time points. (categorical) Distribution adequate for short-term, but not for intermediate-term or long-term. This is based on too few "3" category studies for medium-term and too few " 2" & "3" categories for long-term.

VARIABLE NAME	VARIABLE DEFINITION AND DISTRIBUTION†
Type of Self-Management Support [A = Active (use of behaviorally-oriented techniques), P = Passive (educational materials without personal contact), N = No evidence of self-management support)	Intervention included self-management support or there was no evidence of self-management support. Support was either active or passive. Used only for qualitative analysis (categorical).
Primary Care Clinicians Are Involved (PCP_Involve = yes)	The intervention specified that primary care clinicians be actively involved in decision-making on depression management, rather than delegating decision-making to others after initial referral to collaborative care (dichotomous). **Distribution not adequate for short-term, intermediate-term or long-term based on too few "no" category studies.**
Mental Health Specialists are Involved (MH_Specialty = yes)	The intervention specified that one or more mental health specialists be actively involved in monitoring patients, either directly or through communication with the primary care clinician or care manager, after initial referral to collaborative care. (dichotomous). **Distribution not adequate for short-term, intermediate-term or long-term based on too few "no" category studies.**
Standardized Care Manager Baseline Symptom Assessment (CM_Staff_Base_Sx = yes)**	Dedicated care manager staff conducted assessment of patient symptoms at baseline using a standardized scale. By dedicated, we mean an individual who carried out this function as a defined, discrete job, rather than e.g. a primary care clinician or pharmacist engaged in usual practice. Usually studies also indicated specific training (dichotomous). **Distribution not adequate for short-term, intermediate-term or long-term based on too few "no" category studies.**

VARIABLE NAME	VARIABLE DEFINITION AND DISTRIBUTION†
Standardized Care Manager Follow-up Symptom Assessment *(CM_Staff_F_U_SX = yes)****	Dedicated care manager staff conducted followed up assessments of patient symptoms using a standardized scale. By dedicated, we mean an individual carried out this function as a defined, discrete job. Usually studies also indicated specific training (dichotomous). **Distribution adequate for short-term, but not medium-term or long-term based on too few "no" category studies.**
Care Manager Follow-up of Treatment Adherence *(CM_Staff_F_U_Adh = yes)*****	Dedicated care manager staff F\followed patients proactively for treatment adherence. By dedicated, we mean an individual who carried out this function as a defined, discrete job. Usually studies also indicated specific training (dichotomous). **Distribution not adequate for short-term, intermediate-term or long-term based on too few "no" category studies.**

*CMAssess2 same as *CMAssess* except that the Dietrick article is coded as "yes" rather than "9" for base symtoms
**Same coding as *BaseSx* except that the Dietrick article is coded as "yes" rather than "9"
***Same coding as *DepScale*
****Same coding as *TxAdhere*
†Adequacy of variable distribution is based on having at least three studies with each variable value, see analysis methods. Short-term, medium-term, and long-term refer to time of measurement of effects, see outcome variable definitions. Intervention characteristics that were too prevalent in the sample to be investigated quantitatively and were therefore subjected to qualitative impact analysis are listed in bold.

Table 2: Summary of study design characteristics

Characteristic	Category	n
Study quality	Low risk of bias	18
	Moderate risk of bias	6
	High risk of bias	4
Comparator	Usual care	15
	Usual care: all patients starting antidepressant	12
	Consult-liaison mental health	1
Location	Latin America	1
	United States	23
	Western Europe	4
Setting	Community	8
	Academic	2
	HMO or Veterans Affairs	15
	Mixed	3
Patient recruitment	Systematic screening	11
	Administrative database or pharmacist	6
	Clinician referral	9
	Mixed	2
Major depression	< 75% of patients had MDD	14
	>= 75% of patients had MDD	9
	Unknown	5
Patient population	< 25% ethnic minorities	15
	>= 25% ethnic minorities	7
	Unknown	6
Psychiatric comorbidity	Not excluded systematically	13
	Bipolar disorder, psychosis and substance abuse excluded or triaged to mental health specialist	15

Table 3: Evaluation Design Features Versus Study Effects on Depression Symptoms or Depression Resolution*

Intervention Feature	Response Category	Depression Symptom Effects						Depression Resolution	
		Short-term Effect Size (95% CI)		Medium-term Effect Size (95% CI)		Long-term Effect Size (95% CI)		Relative Risk (95% CI)	
		n		n		n		n	
Number of Practices in the Study (*practice_group*)	Few	5	-0.18 (-0.43, 0.06)	5	-0.08 (-0.38, 0.22)	2	-0.02 (-0.40, 0.35)	5	1.19 (0.90, 1.55)
	Medium	8	-0.33 (-0.50, -0.17)	8	-0.32 (-0.52, -0.12)	4	-0.12 (-0.34, 0.11)	8	1.49 (1.20, 1.84)
	Many	8	-0.28 (-0.46, -0.11)	5	-0.26 (-0.50, -0.01)	4	-0.33 (-0.54, -0.12)	5	1.47 (1.15, 1.88)
Referred to the Study after Screening Only (*type_ref1*)	Yes	7	-0.37 (-0.53, -0.20)	8	-0.33 (-0.52, -0.13)	7	-0.24 (-0.41, -0.07)	6	1.76 (1.44, 2.14)
	No	14	-0.23 (-0.36, -0.10)	10	-0.18 (-0.37, 0.01)	3	-0.07 (-0.36, 0.22)	12	1.24 (1.08, 1.43)*
Referred to the Study by Primary Care Clinicians and on Antidepressant Medications or Willing to Take Them (*type ref2*)	Yes	7	-0.23 (-0.42, -0.03)	8	-0.14 (-0.35, 0.08)	2	-0.08 (-0.46, 0.30)	8	1.24 (1.02, 1.52)
	No	14	-0.31 (-0.44, -0.19)	10	-0.32 (-0.49, -0.15)	8	-0.22 (-0.38, -0.05)	10	1.53 (1.28, 1.82)
Patient Level Randomization (*rand1*)	Yes	13	-0.30 (-0.44, -0.16)	12	-0.27 (-0.44, -0.09)	3	-0.10 (-0.40, 0.19)	11	1.32 (1.11, 1.58)
	No	8	-0.27 (-0.43, -0.10)	6	-0.22 (-0.45, 0.00)	7	-0.23 (-0.41, -0.06)	7	1.53 (1.22, 1.90)
More than 25% of Patients Were Non-White (*minority grp*)	Yes	6	-0.35 (-0.55, -0.14)	7	-0.29 (-0.51, -0.06)	4	-0.16 (-0.39, 0.07)	6	1.50 (1.17, 1.93)
	No	10	-0.24 (-0.41, -0.08)	8	-0.24 (-0.46, -0.02)	6	-0.23 (-0.42, -0.03)	12	1.35 (1.14, 1.61)

* See Table 1 for full variable descriptions.

34

Table 4a: Collaborative Care Intervention Model Feature Effects on Depression Symptoms or Depression Resolution (Initial Variables)*

Collaborative Care Model Intervention Features — Features	Response Category	Depression Symptom Effects								Depression Resolution	
		Short-term		Medium-term		Long-term:				Relative Risk	
		n	Effect Size (95% CI)	n	Effect Size (95% CI)	n	Effect Size (95% CI)			n	(95% CI)
Structured DCM Assessment of Depression Symptoms (Baseline and Followup) and Treatment Adherence (CMAssess)	Yes	15	-0.23 (-0.34, -0.12)	15	-0.20 (-0.33, -0.06)	10	NE			14	1.38 (1.17, 1.62)
	No	6	-0.44 (-0.63, -0.25)	3	-0.53 (-0.83, -0.22)	0	NE			4	1.47 (1.09, 1.98)
Active Self-Management Support (self_manage)	Yes	7	-0.37 (-0.54, -0.20)	8	-0.33 (-0.53, -0.13)	4	-0.30 (-0.51, -0.08)			8	1.64 (1.36, 1.99)*
	No	14	-0.24 (-0.37, -0.11)	10	-0.18 (-0.37, 0.00)	6	-0.12 (-0.31, 0.07)			10	1.24 (1.04, 1.46)
Care Manager Triage to Mental Health (MH_spec)	Yes	7	-0.20 (-0.38, -0.02)	6	-0.14 (-0.38, 0.10)	4	-0.02 (-0.25, 0.20)			5	1.29 (0.98, 1.69)
	No	14	-0.33 (-0.45, -0.20)	12	-0.30 (-0.46, -0.14)	6	-0.29 (-0.45, -0.14)			13	1.44 (1.22, 1.70)
Primary Care Clinician Adjusts Antidepressants	Yes	17	-0.25 (-0.36, -0.13)	14	-0.19 (-0.34, -0.04)	8	-0.18 (-0.35, -0.01)			15	1.34 (1.15, 1.56)
	No	4	-0.44 (-0.66, -0.21)	4	-0.45 (-0.72, -0.19)	2	-0.25 (-0.59, 0.09)			3	1.69 (1.23, 2.33)
Care Managers were predominately medical nurses (CMMed Nurse)	Yes	8	-0.31 (-0.48, -0.15)	9	-0.31 (-0.50, -0.13)	6	-0.28 (-0.45, -0.11)			7	1.60 (1.32, 1.94)
	No	13	-0.26 (-0.40, -0.12)	9	-0.17 (-0.37, 0.03)	4	-0.05 (-0.28, 0.18)			11	1.26 (1.07, 1.49)

Table 4b: Collaborative Care Intervention Model Feature Effects on Depression Symptoms or Depression Resolution (Additional Variables)*

Intervention Feature	Response Category	Depression Symptom Effects						Depression Resolution	
		n	Short-term Effect Size (95% CI)	n	Medium-term Effect Size (95% CI)	n	Long-term Effect Size (95% CI)	n	Relative Risk (95% CI)
Intensity of Intervention Assessment and Follow-Up (*robustness*)	High	11	-0.21 (-0.36, -0.07)	11	-0.19 (-0.36, -0.01)	6	-0.20 (-0.41, 0.01)	11	1.37 (1.13, 1.65)
	Med	4	-0.28 (-0.52, -0.05)	2	-0.17 (-0.55, 0.21)	1	-0.08 (-0.58, 0.41)	2	1.33 (0.89, 1.98)
	Low	6	-0.40 (-0.59, -0.22)	5	-0.42 (-0.67, -0.16)	3	-0.23 (-0.52, 0.07)	5	1.50 (1.14, 1.96)
Classic Collaborative Care Intervention With Long Follow-up (*type_int1*)	Yes	14	-0.29 (-0.42, -0.16)	13	-0.24 (-0.40, -0.07)	5	-0.34 (-0.50, -0.17)*	13	1.44 (1.22, 1.70)
	No	7	-0.27 (-0.46, -0.08)	5	-0.28 (-0.55, -0.02)	5	-0.05 (-0.23, 0.13)	5	1.28 (0.98, 1.68)
Active Patient Follow-up for At Least 16 Weeks (*_16_weeks*)	Yes	17	-0.24 (-0.34, -0.13)*	16	-0.20 (-0.33, -0.07)*	8	-0.22 (-0.39, -0.06)	16	1.38 (1.19, 1.60)
	No	4	-0.52 (-0.75, -0.28)	2	-0.63 (-1.00, -0.26)	2	-0.08 (-0.42, 0.26)	2	1.59 (1.04, 2.43)

* See Table 1 for full variable descriptions.

Table 5: Relationship between Qualitative Impact Variable and Effects on Depression Symptoms and Resolution*

Intervention Feature	Response Category	Depression Symptoms						Depression Resolution	
		Short-term: Effect Size (95% CI)	n	Intermediate: Effect Size (95% CI)	n	Long-term: Effect Size (95% CI)	n	Relative Risk (95% CI)	n
	High Impact (1)	-0.40 (-0.56, -0.24)	8	-0.42 (-0.59, -0.25)	9	-0.37 (-0.56, -0.18)	4	1.71 (1.47, 1.99)	8
	Medium (2)	-0.26 (-0.44, -0.08)	6	-0.15 (-0.39, 0.08)	4	-0.08 (-0.47, 0.31)	1	1.35 (1.12, 1.63)	5
Overall Intervention Impact (*impact*)	Low (3)	-0.30 (-0.59, -0.01)	3	-0.11 (-0.58, 0.36)	1	-0.10 (-0.39, 0.18)	2	1.24 (0.88, 1.76)	2
	Little or no impact (4)	-0.07 (-0.30, 0.16)*	4	0.02 (-0.25, 0.29)*	4	-0.01 (-0.28, 0.25)*	3	0.91 (0.70, 1.18)*	3

*See Methods section for full description of the impact variable.

37

Table 6: Qualitative Impact Analysis Table of Intervention Features*

Studies Ranked by Impact	Type of Self-Management Support A = Active (use of behaviorally-oriented techniques) P = Passive (educational materials without personal contact) N = No evidence of self-management support	Primary Care Clinicians Actively Involved in Patient Management (PCP_Involve) Y= Yes N= No	Mental Health Specialists Actively Involved in Patient Management (MH_Specialty) Y= Yes N= No	CM Baseline Assessment of Patient Symptoms with Standardized Scale (CM_Staff_Base_Sx) Y= Yes N= No	CM Follow-up Assessment of Symptoms with Standardized Scale (CM_Stff_F_U_Sx) Y= Yes N= No	CM Follow-up Assessment of Treatment Adherence (CM_Stff_F_U_Adh) Y= Yes N= No	Intervention included at least 16 weeks of active patient follow-up (_16_weeks) Y= Yes N= No	Overall Impact (impact) 1= High 2 = Medium 3 = Low 4 = Little or None
Araya, 2003	A	Y	Y	Y	Y	Y	N	1
Katon, 1995	A	Y	Y	Y	Y	Y	Y	1
Katon, 1996	A	Y	Y	Y	Y	Y	Y	1
Katon, 1999	A	Y	Y	N	Y	Y	Y	1
Katon, 2004	A	Y	Y	Y	Y	Y	Y	1
Katzelnick, 2000	P	Y	Y	Y	Y	Y	Y	1
Simon, 2004	A	Y	Y	Y	Y	Y	Y	1
Unutzer, 2002***	A	Y	Y	Y	Y	Y	Y	1
Wells, 2000	A	Y	Y	Y	N	Y	Y	1
Bruce, 2004	A	Y	Y	Y	Y	Y	Y	2
Dietrich, 2004	A	Y	Y	Y	Y	Y	Y	2
Hunkeler, 2000	A	Y	Y	N	N	Y	Y	2

38

Studies Ranked by Impact	Type of Self-Management Support	Primary Care Clinicians Actively Involved in Patient Management (PCP_Involve)	Mental Health Specialists Actively Involved in Patient Management (MH_Specialty)	CM Baseline Assessment of Patient Symptoms with Standardized Scale (CM_Staff_Base_Sx)	CM Follow-up Assessment of Symptoms with Standardized Scale (CM_Stff_F_U_Sx)	CM Follow-up Assessment of Treatment Adherence (CM_Stff_F_U_Adh)	Intervention included at least 16 weeks of active patient follow-up (_16_weeks)	Overall Impact (impact)
	A = Active (use of behaviorally-oriented techniques) P = Passive (educational materials without personal contact) N = No evidence of self-management support	Y= Yes N= No	Y= Yes N= No	Y= Yes N= No	Y= Yes N= No	Y= Yes N= No	Y= Yes N= No	1= High 2 = Medium 3 = Low 4 = Little or None
Oslin, 2003**	A	Y	Y	Y	Y	Y	Y	2
Peveler, 1999	P	Y	Y	Y	N	N	N	2
Rost, 2001	A	Y	N	Y	Y	Y	Y	2
Simon, 2000	N	Y	Y	Y	Y	Y	Y	2
Datto, 2003	N	Y	Y	Y	Y	Y	Y	3
Fortney, 2006**	A	Y	Y	Y	Y	Y	Y	3
Hedrick, 2003**	P	Y	Y	Y	Y	Y	Y	3
Waterreus, 2004	A	N	?	Y	Y	Y	N	3
20 90% = 18								
80% = 16	A = 15	Y = 19	Y = ?18	Y = 18	Y = 17	Y = 19	Y = 17	
70% = 14								
Adler, 2004	P	Y	Y	Y	Y	Y	Y	4

Studies Ranked by Impact	Type of Self-Management Support A = Active (use of behaviorally-oriented techniques) P = Passive (educational materials without personal contact) N = No evidence of self-management support	Primary Care Clinicians Actively Involved in Patient Management (PCP_Involve) Y= Yes N= No	Mental Health Specialists Actively Involved in Patient Management (MH_Specialty) Y= Yes N= No	CM Baseline Assessment of Patient Symptoms with Standardized Scale (CM_Staff_Base_Sx) Y= Yes N= No	CM Follow-up Assessment of Symptoms with Standardized Scale (CM_Stff_F_U_Sx) Y= Yes N= No	CM Follow-up Assessment of Treatment Adherence (CM_Stff_F_U_Adh) Y= Yes N= No	Intervention included at least 16 weeks of active patient follow-up (_16_weeks) Y= Yes N= No	Overall Impact (impact) 1= High 2 = Medium 3 = Low 4 = Little or None
Brook, 2005	P	N	N	N	Y	Y	N	4
Cappocia, 2004	N	Y	Y	Y	Y	Y	Y	4
Dobscha, 2006**	P	Y	Y	Y	Y	Y	N	4
Finley, 2003	N	Y	Y	Y	Y	Y	Y	4
Mann, 1998	N	Y	N	Y	N	Y	Y	4
Rickles, 2005	N	N	N	N	N	Y	N	4
Swindle, 2003**	N	Y	Y	Y	Y	Y	N	4
8								
90% = 7.2								
80% = 6.4	A = 0	Y = 6	Y = 5	Y = 6	Y = 6	Y = 8	Y = 4	
70% = 5.6								

* See Methods section for full description of the impact variable. See Table 1 for full descriptions of the remaining variables. **VA studies. ***Had a VA site.

Table 7. Qualitative Comorbidity Ranked by Overall Impact*

Study	Proportion with Major Depressive Disorder (MDD)	Proportion Non-White (Minority)	Exclude Substance Abuse? (E_SA) 1= yes 0= No	Exclude Dementia? (E_Dementia) 1= yes 0= No	Exclude PTSD? (E_PTSD) 1= yes 0= No	Exclude Anxiety? (E_Anxiety) 1= yes 0= No	Exclude Psychosis? (E_Psychosis) 1= yes 0= No	Exclude Bipolar Disorder? (E_BD) 1= yes 0= No	Overall Impact 1= High 2= Medium 3= Low 4= Little or None
Araya	1	1	1	0	0	0	1	1	1
Katon 1995	0.419	No Data	1	1	9	0	1	1	1
Katon 1996	0.424	0.13	1	1	9	0	1	1	1
Katon 1999	0.798	0.17	1	9	9	0	1	1	1
Katon 2004	0.62	0.25	1	0	0	0	1	1	1
Katzelnick	1	0.17	1	9	0	0	1	1	1
Simon 2004	0.59	0.2	0	0	0	0	1	1	1
Wells	0.563	0.43	0	1	0	0	0	0	1
Unutzer	0.69	0.245	1	1	0	0	0	1	2
Bruce	0.662	0.33	0	1	0	0	0	0	2
Dietrich	0.79	0.167	1	0	1	0	1	1	2
Hunkeler	.	0.37	1	0	0	0	1	1	2
Oslin	0.688	0.55	0	1	1	0	1	1	2
Peveler	0.49	No Data	0	1	0	0	0	0	2
Rost	0.774	0.157	1	9	9	9	1	1	2
Simon	.	No Data	1	1	0	0	1	1	2
Datto	0.847	0.2	1	9	9	9	1	1	3
Fortney	0.82	0.253	1	1	1	0	1	1	3
Hedrick	0.944	0.2	1	1	1	0	0	No Data	3
Waterreus	0.24	No Data	No Data	0	0	0	0	No Data	3
Adler	0.76	0.276	1	1	0	0	1	1	4
Brook	.	0.01	0	0	0	0	0	0	4
Cappocia	0.41	0.22	1	0	0	0	1	0	4
Dobscha	0.49	0.05	0	1	0	0	0	1	4
Finley	.	No Data	1	0	0	0	0	1	4
Mann	0.82	No Data	0	0	0	0	0	1	4
Rickles	.	0.08	0	0	0	0	1	1	4
Swindle	0.88	0.142	1	1	9	9	1	1	4

* See Methods section for full description of the impact variable. See Table 1 for full descriptions of the remaining variables.

Table 8. Design Features Ranked by Overall Impact*

Study	Overall Impact (impact) 1= High 2 = Medium 3 = Low 4 = Little or None	Number of Practices (practice group) Small = 1 to 2 Medium = 3 to 10 Large >10	Type of Randomization 1 = Patient Level 2 = Practice Level 3 = Provider Level	Type of referral 1 = Referred by PCP and on medications or willing to take medications 2 = Referred by PCP or screened and referred 3 = On medications 4 = Screened
Araya	1	M	1	4
Katon 1995	1	S	1	1
Katon 1996	1	S	1	1
Katon 1999	1	M	1	1
Katon 2004	1	M	1	1
Katzelnick	1	L	3	4
Simon 2004	1	M	1	3
Unutzer	1	L	2	4
Wells	1	community	1	4
Bruce	2	L	2	4
Dietrich	2	L	2	1
Hunkeler	2	S	1	1
Oslin	2	M	3	4
Peveler	2	L	1	3
Rost	2	L	2	4
Simon	2	M	1	3
Datto	3	L	2	2
Fortney	3	M	2	4
Hedrick	3	M	2	2
Waterreus	3	L	1	2
Adler	4	M	1	4
Brook	4	community	1	3
Cappocia	4	S	1	1
Dobscha	4	M	3	4
Finley	4	S	1	1
Mann	4	L	1	2
Rickles	4	Community	1	3
Swindle	4	S	2	4

* See Methods section for full description of the impact variable. See Table 1 for full descriptions of the remaining variables.

Table 9: Understanding Self-Management Support

Studies Ranked by Impact	Type of Self-Management Support	Type of Patient Intervention		
	A = Active (use of behaviorally-oriented techniques) P = Passive (educational materials without personal contact) N = No evidence of self-management support			
Araya, 2003	A	Modality:	Psychoeducational intervention group	
		Delivered by:	Social workers and nurses	
		Content:	Depression assessment Treatment options	
		Theory:	Problem-solving techniques Scheduling positive activities Basic cognitive and relapse-prevention techniques	
		Quantity:	7 weekly sessions and 2 booster sessions	
		Others Involved:	Structured pharmacotherapy program with PCP if severe depression after 6 weeks	
		Materials:	Manual with examples and exercises	
Katon, 1995	A	Modality:	Psychiatry visits	
		Delivered by:	Psychiatrist	
		Content:	Depression assessment Understanding antidepressant action and side effects Review of stressful life events	
		Theory:	No formal psychotherapy	
		Quantity:	2 to 4 visits with psychiatrist	
		Others Involved:	PCP visits alternated with psychiatrist visits	
		Materials:	Booklet on biology of depression and how antidepressants work Booklet on simple cognitive-behavioral techniques for managing depression Video with doctor-patient vignettes Questionnaire to motivate active patient role	

43

Studies Ranked by Impact	Type of Self-Management Support	Type of Patient Intervention		
	A = Active (use of behaviorally-oriented techniques) P = Passive (educational materials without personal contact) N = No evidence of self-management support			
		Modality:	Psychotherapy	
		Delivered by:	Psychologist	
		Content:	Depression assessment Antidepressant assessment	
		Theory:	Therapeutic techniques based on social cognitive theory and social learning theory models Sessions 1-4: education, skills training, homework assignments or behavioral experiments to improve mood and facilitate generalization of skills to daily life Sessions 5-6 (optional): skills training in assertion, problem-solving communications in conflictual situations, and relaxation training	
		Quantity:	4 to 6 direct contacts followed by 4 telephone contacts	
		Others Involved:	Optional referral to psychiatrist for nonresponding patients	
		Materials:	Booklet on biology of depression and how antidepressants work Booklet on simple cognitive-behavioral techniques for managing depression; "I can If I Want To" Video with doctor-patient vignettes	
Katon, 1996	A			
		Modality:	Psychiatry visits	
		Delivered by:	Psychiatrist	
		Content:	Depression assessment Review of stressful life events Review of medication adherence and side effects Review of medical, family, and social history	
		Theory:	Optional psychotherapy for patients with severe psychosocial stressors	
		Quantity:	2 sessions with psychiatrist with additional visits based on clinical response—brief telephone call between visits	
Katon, 1999	A	Others Involved:	PCP encouraged to discuss patient reactions/questions regarding educational materials	

Studies Ranked by Impact	Type of Self-Management Support	Type of Patient Intervention	
	A = Active (use of behaviorally-oriented techniques) P = Passive (educational materials without personal contact) N = No evidence of self-management support		
		Materials:	Book and videotape addressing biology of depression, antidepressdant medications, psychotherapy, and active self-management
Katon, 2004	A	Modality:	Pathways case management intervention—antidepressant medications and/or PST-PC
		Delivered by:	Depression Clinical Specialist Nurse
		Content:	Enhanced education
			Support for antidepressant medication
		Theory:	Problem-solving treatment in primary care (PST-PC)
		Quantity:	Initial visit, step 1—twice monthly contacts for 10-12 weeks, step2—bimonthly contacts for 8-12 weeks, step 3—referral to mental health system for longer–term follow-up if needed, continuation phase—monthly contacts or groups if significant decrease in symptoms
		Others Involved:	Optional psychiatric consultation, collaboration with PCP
		Materials:	None specified
Katzelnick, 2000	P	Modality:	Telephone-based treatment coordination
		Delivered by:	Treatment coordinators some with mental health background
		Content:	Depression assessment
			Treatment adherence and medication effects
		Theory:	No formal psychotherapy
		Quantity:	PCP visits: initial, follow-up at 1, 3, 6, 10 weeks, then every 10 weeks; treatment coordinator

45

Studies Ranked by Impact	Type of Self-Management Support	Type of Patient Intervention	
	A = Active (use of behaviorally-oriented techniques) P = Passive (educational materials without personal contact) N = No evidence of self-management support		contacts: at 2, 10 weeks, and if needed at 18, 30, 42 weeks
		Others Involved:	PCP, Psychiatric consultation encourage if no response to treatment at 10 weeks or if complicated depression
		Materials:	Booklet on "Depression isn't Just a Mental Problem," video, RHYTHMS depression ecucation program if appropriate to support antidepressant use
		Modality:	Psychotherapy (telephone-based)
		Delivered by:	Psychotherapists
		Content:	Depression assessment Antidepressant use and adverse effects
		Theory:	CBT program
		Quantity:	CBT: 1—motivation, 2 to 4—increasing pleasant and rewarding activities, 5-7—identifying challenges and distancing from negative thoughts, 8—self-care plan
		Others Involved:	Care managers: mental health clinicians with bachelor's or master's degrees (care management program in addition to psychotherapy)
Simon, 2004	A	Materials:	Detailed care management workbook emphasizing activation, addressing negative thought, developing self-care plan
		Modality:	IMPACT intervention—antidepressant medications and/or PST-PC
		Delivered by:	Nurses or psychologists trained as depression care managers
		Content:	Depression assessment
		Theory:	Problem-solving treatment in primary care (PST-PC)
		Quantity:	PST-PC: 6-8 sessions; care manager contacts every other week during the acute phase and monthly if reduction in symptoms up to 12 months
		Others Involved:	Psychiatrist contact if lack of response or diagnostic challenge; PCP
Unutzer, 2002	A	Materials:	Video, booklet

46

Studies Ranked by Impact	Type of Self-Management Support	Type of Patient Intervention	
	A = Active (use of behaviorally-oriented techniques) P = Passive (educational materials without personal contact) N = No evidence of self-management support		
Wells, 2000	A	Modality:	Psychotherapy or antidepressant medication support
		Delivered by:	QI meds: Nurse specialists QI therapy: Psychotherapists
		Content:	QI meds: depression assessment, support adherence QI therapy: individual and group CBT
		Theory:	CBT
		Quantity:	Initial visit for assessment, education, and activation QI meds: monthly contacts QI therapy: 12 to 16 sessions
		Others Involved:	Not specified
		Materials:	Videos and pamphlets
Bruce, 2004	A	Modality:	Treatment management
		Delivered by:	Depression care managers
		Content:	Depression assessment Treatment adherence and medication adverse side effects PCP could recommend interpersonal psychotherapy if patient declined medication
		Theory:	Not specified
		Quantity:	At scheduled intervals or when clinically necessary—frequency not specified
		Others Involved:	Collaborated with PCP
		Materials:	Not specified
Dietrich, 2004	A	Modality:	Telephone-based care management
		Delivered by:	Care managers—most with backgrounds in primary care or mental health nursing
		Content:	Overcoming barriers to adherence Supported self-management practices (e.g., exercise, social activities)
		Theory:	Not specified

47

Studies Ranked by Impact	Type of Self-Management Support	Type of Patient Intervention		
	A = Active (use of behaviorally-oriented techniques) P = Passive (educational materials without personal contact) N = No evidence of self-management support			
		Quantity:	Initial contact, contacts monthly thereafter or as needed	
		Others Involved:	Intervention clinician	
		Materials:	Not specified	
		Modality:	Telehealth care	
		Delivered by:	Primary care nurses	
		Content:	Antidepressant adherence, side effects, questions Emotional support to find pleasurable activities and to be more active Support for behavior plan	
		Theory:	Not specified	
Hunkeler, 2000	A	Quantity:	Weeks 1-2: 1 to 2 calls per week; weeks 3-8: 1 call per week; weeks 9-16: 1 call every other week	
		Others Involved:	Peer support in addition to nurse telehealth care in 35% of intervention patients	
		Materials:	Not specified	
		Modality:	Telephone disease management	
		Delivered by:	Behanioral health specialist (nurses with behavioral health experience)	
		Content:	Depression assessment Treatment adherence and adverse effects Education and motivation support	
		Theory:	Not specified	
Oslin, 2003	A	Quantity:	Calls at 1, 3, 6, 9, 12, 18, and 24 weeks after initial assessment	
		Others Involved:	PCP	
		Materials:	Not specified for depression; workbook for alcohol intervention	
		Modality:	Drug counseling	
Peveler, 1999	P	Delivered by:	Primary care nurses	
		Content:	Education—depression, self-help, treatment adherence	

48

Studies Ranked by Impact	Type of Self-Management Support	Type of Patient Intervention	
	A = Active (use of behaviorally-oriented techniques) P = Passive (educational materials without personal contact) N = Nc evidence of self-management support		
		Theory:	No formal psychotherapy
		Quantity:	At weeks 2 and 8
		Others Involved:	Not specified
		Materials:	Information leaflet
		Modality:	Pharmacotherapy and/or psychotherapy
		Delivered by:	Nurses
		Content:	Depression assessment Education about treatments Supported activation/engagement
		Theory:	Not specifed
		Quantity:	Average of 5.2 contacts during the first 8 weeks after index visit
		Others Involved:	PCP, access to specialty care psychotherapy
Rost, 2001	A	Materials:	AHCPR pamphlet
		Modality:	Care management (1 of 2 interventions)
		Delivered by:	Care managers
		Content:	Antidpressant use, side effects Depression assessment General support
		Theory:	No specific psychotherapeutic content
		Quantity:	Brief initial call followed by 2 calls at 8 and 16 weeks
		Others Involved:	PCP
Simon, 2000	N	Materials:	Not specified
Datto, 2003	N	Modality:	Telephone disease management
		Delivered by:	Nurses

49

Studies Ranked by Impact	Type of Self-Management Support	Type of Patient Intervention	
	A = Active (use of behaviorally-oriented techniques) P = Passive (educational materials without personal contact) N = No evidence of self-management support		
		Content:	Education topics: depression, treatment options, coping skills, risk factors, suicide prevention, reinforcing followup Depression assessment Treatment adherence
		Theory:	Not specified
		Quantity:	Followup contact at least every 3 weeks; formal assessment at baseline, 6, 12, and 16 weeks
		Others Involved:	PCP
		Materials:	Not specified
		Modality:	Telemedicine-based collaborative care (stepped care)
		Delivered by:	Nurses
		Content:	Education' Activation and barrier assessment/resolution activities Depression assessment Treatment adherence and side effects
		Theory:	Psychotherapy was available but not facilitated
		Quantity:	Followup: acute—every 2 weeks, watchful waiting or continuation—every 4 weeks for up to 12 months
		Others Involved:	PCP, pharmacist
Fortney, 2006	A	Materials:	Pamphlet and website

50

Studies Ranked by Impact	Type of Self-Management Support	Type of Patient Intervention	
	A = Active (use of behaviorally-oriented techniques) P = Passive (educational materials without personal contact) N = No evidence of self-management support		
Hedrick, 2003	P	Modality:	Collaborative care (treatment options: antidepressant medication initiation or adjustment, CBT, scheduling with psychologist or psychiatrist, mental health specialty care)
		Delivered by:	CBT: Psychologist or social worker
		Content:	Encourage adherence
			Address treatment barriers
			Depression assessment
		Theory:	CBT
		Quantity:	CBT: 6 sessions
		Others Involved:	Team: clinical psychologist, psychiatrist, social workers, psychology technician
		Materials:	Video and workbook
Waterreus, 2004	A	Modality:	Multifaceted package of care
		Delivered by:	Community psychiatric nurse (CPN)
		Content:	Depression assessment
			Education
			Psychological interventions: 94% of intervention patients
			Pharmacotherapy: 66% of intervention patients
		Theory:	Personal supportive therapy, behaviour therapy and relaxation, family and marital work, bereavement counseling
		Quantity:	Weekly visits over 3 months and contact phone number
		Others Involved:	GP
		Materials:	Not specified
Adler, 2004	P	Modality:	Antidepressant medication support
		Delivered by:	Pharmacist
		Content:	Medication adherence
			General social support

51

Studies Ranked by Impact	Type of Self-Management Support	Type of Patient Intervention	
	A = Active (use of behaviorally-oriented techniques) P = Passive (educational materials without personal contact) N = No evidence of self-management support		
	P	Theory:	No formal psychotherapy
		Quantity:	Contacts at 2,4,6,8 weeks and 6,9,12,18 months
		Others Involved:	Not specified
		Materials:	Not specified
Brook, 2005	P	Modality:	Antidepressant medication support
		Delivered by:	Pharmacist
		Content:	"a list of important themes" not specified
		Theory:	No formal psychotherapy
		Quantity:	3 coaching contacts
		Others Involved:	Not specified
		Materials:	Video
Cappocia, 2004	N	Modality:	Collaborative care
		Delivered by:	Pharmacist
		Content:	Depression assessment
			Antidepressant concerns addressed
			Support and education
			Antidepressant medication adjustments and side effects management
			Facilitation of mental health provider appointments
		Theory:	No formal psychotherapy
		Quantity:	Weeks 1-4—weekly calls, weeks 5-12—calls every 2 weeks, months 3-12—calls every other month
		Others Involved:	PCP , psychiatrist
		Materials:	Not specified
Dobscha, 2006	P	Modality:	Decision support
		Delivered by:	Depression decision support nurse care manager

Studies Ranked by Impact	Type of Self-Management Support A = Active (use of behaviorally-oriented techniques) P = Passive (educational materials without personal contact) N = No evidence of self-management support		Type of Patient Intervention
		Content:	Education--explore barriers, treatment adherence, encourage communication with providers
		Theory:	No formal psychotherapy
		Quantity:	1 early telephone contact
		Others Involved:	Psychiatrist
		Materials:	Supplemental educational materials
		Modality:	Drug therapy management (feature of collaborative care)
		Delivered by:	Pharmacist
		Content:	Antidepressant adherence and adverse effects, titrate medications Depression assessment Other social and medical factors
		Theory:	No formal psychotherapy
		Quantity:	Calls at weeks 1,2,4,10, and 16, clinic visits at weeks 6 and 24
		Others Involved:	Not specified
Finley, 2003	N	Materials:	Not specified
		Modality:	Monitoring (1 of 2 interventions)
		Delivered by:	Practice nurses
		Content:	Content of interview recorded as follows: monitoring change in mental health, encouraging compliance, providing education, facilitating social intervention
		Theory:	No formal psychotherapy
		Quantity:	8 hours per patient over 4 months re commended
		Others Involved:	GP
Mann, 1998	N	Materials:	Not specified
		Modality:	Telemonitoring of antidepressant use
		Delivered by:	Pharmacist
Rickles, 2005	N	Content:	Medication adherence and adverse effects

Studies Ranked by Impact	Type of Self-Management Support	Type of Patient Intervention	
	A = Active (use of behaviorally-oriented techniques) P = Passive (educational materials without personal contact) N = No evidence of self-management support		Patient concerns
		Theory:	No formal psychotherapy
		Quantity:	3 monthly telephone calls
		Others Involved:	Not specified
		Materials:	Not specified
		Modality:	Monitoring
		Delivered by:	Mental health clinical nurse specialists
		Content:	Depression assessment Review side effects Encourage compliance with antidepressants
		Theory:	No formal psychotherapy
		Quantity:	Contacts at 2 weeks, 1 month, and 2 months after initial contact
		Others Involved:	PCP, referral to mental health clinic if patient unable to take antidepressant medication for CBT or more complex medication regimen
Swindle, 2003	N	Materials:	Not specified

54

Appendix A

Study	Organization (practices)	n	Study Quality		Risk of bias
			Analysis (follow-up rate)	Blinding outcomes assessment	
Adler et al., 2004	Academic and community (9 practices; 53 clinicians)	507	Intent-to-treat (3 months, 73%; 6 months, 76%)	Yes	Low
Araya et al., 2003	3 Clinics, Santiago, Chile (clinicians, NS)	240	Intent-to-treat (3 months, 88%; 6 months, 88%)	Yes	Low
Brook et al., 2005	General practice, The Netherlands (19 community pharmacists; clinicians not involved)	135	Intent-to-treat (3 months, 88%; 6 months, 81%)	Yes	Moderate
Bruce et al., 2004	(20 Community practices; number of clinicians, NS)	598	Intent-to-treat (4 months, 82%; 8 months, 76%; 12 months, 69%)	Yes	Low
Capoccia et al., 2004	Academic family practice clinic (20 staff physicians; 18 trainees; 4 Physician Assistants)	74	Intent-to-treat (3 months, 96%; 6 months, 95%; 9 months, 95%; 12 months, 93%)	Yes	Low
Datto et al., 2003	University-affiliated (35 practices; 151 clinicians)	61	Completers (6 months, 86%)	No	High
Dietrich et al., 2004	5 Health care organizations (60 practices; 226 clinicians)	405	Intent-to-treat (4 months, 82%; 8 months, 76%; 12 months, 69%)	Yes	Low
Dobscha et al., 2006	Veterans Affairs (5 practices; 41 clinicians)	375	Intent-to-treat (6 months, 84%; 12 months, 85%)	Yes	Low
Finley et al., 2003	Staff model HMO (1 practice; 30 clinicians)	125	Completers (6 months, 67%)	Yes	High
Fortney et al., 2006	Veterans Affairs: community clinics (7 clinics)	395	Intent-to-treat (6 months, 91%; 12 months, 85%)	Partially met	Moderate
Hedrick et al., 2003	Veterans Affairs (4 firms; 89 clinicians)	354	Intent-to-treat (3 months, 92%; 9 months, 92%)	Yes	Low

Study	Organization (practices)	n	Study Quality Analysis (follow-up rate)	Blinding outcomes assessment	Risk of bias
Hunkeler et al., 2000	Staff model HMO (2 practices; 100 clinicians)	302	Completers (6 weeks, 90%; 6 months, 85%)	NS	Moderate
Katon et al., 1995	Staff model HMO (1 practice; 22 clinicians)	217	Completers (4 months, 89%; 7 months, 85%)	Yes	Moderate
Katon et al., 1996	Staff model HMO (1 practice; 22 clinicians)	153	Intent-to-treat (4 months, 84%; 7 months, 76%)	Yes	Low
Katon et al., 1999	Staff model HMO (4 practices; 73 clinicians)	228	Intent-to-treat (3 months, 85%; 6 months, 84%; 28 months, 75%)	Yes	Low
Katon et al., 2004	Staff model HMO (9 practices)	329	(3 months, 93%; 6 months, 89%; 12 months, 88%)	Yes	Low
Katzelnick et al., 2000	3 HMOs (practices, NS; 163 clinicians)	407	Intent-to-treat (3 months, 94%; 6 months, 94%; 12 months, 93%)	Yes	Low
Mann et al., 1998	General practice, (19 practices)	419	Intent-to-treat (4 months, 92%)	No	High
Oslin et al., 2003	Veterans Affairs (4 practices; 37 clinicians)	97	Intent-to-treat (4 months, 76%)	Yes	Low
Peveler et al., 1999	General practice, (28 practices; 47 clinicians)	213	Intent-to-treat (6 weeks, 97%; 3 months, 96%)	Yes	Low
Rickles et al., 2005	(14 Community pharmacists; 60 clinicians)	63	Intent-to-treat (3 months, 95%)	Yes	Moderate
Rost et al., 2001	(12 Community practices; 24 clinicians) Mixed (8 systems;	479	Intent-to-treat (6 months, 90%; 24 months, 67%)	Yes	Low
Simon et al., 2000	Staff model HMO (5 practices; 40–50 clinicians)	613	Intent-to-treat (3 months, 97%; 6 months, 96%; 60 months, 73%)	Yes	Low
Simon et al., 2004	Staff model HMO (7 practices)	600	Intent-to-treat (6 months, 89%; 18 months, 85%)	Yes	Low

| Study | Organization (practices) | n | Study Quality | | |
			Analysis (follow-up rate)	Blinding outcomes assessment	Risk of bias
Swindle et al., 2003	Veterans Affairs (2 firms; 23 clinicians; 100 trainees)	268	Completers (3 months, 92%; 6 months, 83%)	NS	High
Unutzer et al., 2002	18 practices; 367 clinicians)	1801	Intent-to-treat (3 months, 90%; 6 months, 87%; 12 months, 83%)	Yes	Low
Waterreus et al., 1994	General practice, London, UK (practices, NS; 25 clinicians)	96	Completers (3 months, NS; 6 months, NS; 12 months, NS)	Yes	Moderate
Wells et al., 2000	Staff model and network-managed care (46 practices; 181 clinicians)	1356	Intent-to-treat (6 months, 85%; 12 months, 83%)	Yes	Low

Appendix B. Peer Review Table--Evidence Synthesis For Determining Key Features of Effective Depression Interventions

Section of Report	Actual Comments	Changes
All	Should be reviewed and perhaps rewritten for clarity. Sentence structure difficult to interpret i.e. page 22 first sentence. I had to read this sentence multiple times before I understood intent. (Correlations for evaluation features showed that.......) Consider more sentences but each much shorter.	Re-written and clarified.
Conclusions	"I also do see much of an emphasis that these results are really related to major depression and not subsyndromal or minor depression."	Added
Executive Summary	Suggest that clearly state at the top of page 6 that the outcomes of interest here are related to depression outcome and not other outcomes (HRQoL or mortality), and that analysis relating to comorbidities was limited to psychiatric comorbidities.	On pages 6 and 7, we now clarify that we did aim to look for medical comorbidities, but the studies did not support it. We also clarify that our impact measure reviewed adherence, satisfaction, and functioning. We provide additional detail on these issues later in the document.
Executive Summary	I found the summary to be a bit difficult to read, especially if I had been unfamiliar with the field. Defining terms such as "collaborative care model", "chronic illness model", "Patient self management", etc. early on would help the reader. They are defined later in the work but only after they have been used many times. Page 6: would suggest a word replacement for one of the "interventions". It would read better.	More definition is now up front. Page 6 sentence fixed.
Executive Summary	"Research questions didn't address any comorbid medical conditions, which might be very important in a primary care focus (page 6 Primary and Secondary Research Questions)."	Excellent idea, but studies did not include information on medical comorbidities. We have added this to our aims (we did intend to look at this) and limitations.
Executive Summary	"Page 1 gives no reference for their statement "without implementation of organizational changes in primary care practices less than half of patient found to have major depression complete minimally adequate medications or psychotherapy." "	We now reference this statement.
Executive Summary	"The paper recommends elements of patient activation despite that they only reviewed studies with a patient directed component. Page 5 states: "We did not review studies that only sought to change primary care clinician behavior, without an additional patient-directed component." Page 7 concludes "patient self-management support as the single statistically significant intervention characteristic associated with improved depression symptoms and depression resolution"---but it seems they excluded all studies without a patient directed component."	We now clarify with examples that the requirement for a patient directed component was not aimed at patient self-management support, but rather at excluding studies focused only on provider-level interventions such as education or decision support. As shown in our tables, many studies did not include active self-management support.

58

Section	Comment	Response
Introduction	Objectives and scope are clearly described	
Introduction	Suggest a better term [see page 9] than 'mild' major depression, which sounds like a non sequitur; perhaps major depression of lesser severity, which is less likely to be misinterpreted by the reader as minor depression, which is a less compelling clinical and policy target and not the focus of discussion here.	Changed.
Introduction	Suggest transparency would argue for an explicit identification [e.g., personal communication] of the second study referenced at the top of page 10; I suspect the study in question is an analysis from the PRISMe trial.	It isn't PRISMe; it's an AHRQ review just released and is now referenced (Butler).
Introduction	I would take issue with the wording "to fill in for the required depression treatment support functions" at the bottom of page 12. This describes tasks in a strictly co-located rather than collaborative model, and I would recommend something like "to fill in gaps" (in usual practice) or "to support."	Changed.
Introduction	The goals and objectives of the review are clearly stated. The approach to literature review and data synthesis is of interest and compelling.	
Introduction	"This is a little misleading since severe depression is not often included." Regarding statement of collaborative care and major depression with mild symptoms (bottom of page 9)	Changed.
Introduction	"The term nurse is not always right. Not all care management uses nurses" Regarding Fig 2 (page 12)	Changed.
Introduction	"The range of severity also varies from subsyndromal and up though most exclude complex patients" Addition at top of page 14--variation in studies	Changed.
Introduction	"On page 15, it appears that the authors used the Williams review 2007 as the basis for their paper. It appears that the Williams study focused on 28 studies. How does what the authors did differ from what Williams already did?"	We have added to our explanations on this.
Limitations	"Not mentioned is the extensive selection bias that occurs in these studies in regards to participation. Even the studies that use screening exclude many patients or many to no agree to participate. Therefore we don't really know how well these models can be applied to the general population in a primary care practice."	Added.
Methods	Methods are clearly described	
Methods	No related studies overlooked	
Methods	Page 18: for the short, medium, and long effect size groups, were those that showed effects in more than one group given greater weight on impact analysis?	See above re more information on the impact variable; yes, the impact variable considered how durable and consistent the improvement was.
Methods	Not aware of any related depression studies that have been overlooked	

Methods	"The way I read the exclusion criteria, it isn't clear why the prisme study wasn't included. Krahn, etal. Otherwise the exclusion needs to say that the control group was always usual care"	Added usual care
Methods	"Of the 1464 studies identified, why did only 28 get analyzed? Do the authors feel that the 28 studies, less than half of which were published in the last 5 years, provide an adequate basis to make generalizations, or are the numbers so small that the take home message should be to just to fund more studies? Of the 28 studies analyzed, what were the controls? The studies demonstrate that depression improves with a primary care clinician, a mental health clinician, a care manager, patient self-involvement, but compared to what? Compared to no care? Compared to just a primary clinician alone? Compared to a mental health clinician? Compared to having both primary care and mental health clinicians and no care manager? Compared to all of the above but no patient involvement?"	The article drop-off seen here is typical of evidence review. See Fig. 1 for exclusion reasons. However, we have included more on this under limitations. Actually, 28 randomized trials on a single type of intervention is a much greater number than is available for many or even most quality improvement interventions. Re controls, we have clarified throughout that the comparison is to usual care.
Methods	With respect to any overlooked studies: "Defer to other subject matter experts"	
Methods	VHA program is primary care-mental health integration [page 15; it is often reversed in common usage but technically mental health-primary care in VA is the placement of medical support in outpatient psychiatric venues]. The Uniform Mental Health Services Package is VHA Handbook 1160.01 for your reference.	Switched and referenced.
Results	No bias in synthesis of the evidence	
Results	I would consider adding a statement to the limitation section, which your statistician feels is appropriate, about the possible relationship between the number of categories for analytic variables, misclassification bias between the categories, and the results presented. In other words, comment on reproducibility/robustness given these categories.	Added.

Results	Are the analyzed interventions unique to PC/MH? Page 17 defines care management as: "abstracted features such as : coordination and communication among providers, patient education, monitoring sxs and adherence to Rx Plans, self management support, and psychological Rx." All of the above seem components of any good treatment plan. Would they have the same impact and effect on any type of disease management program? Individual intervention features were analyzed in the study. Could combinations of interventional variables and their impact yield additional information? Most/Many of the analyzed studies had additional staff support. Could the same clinical effect have been realized by lowering PC panel size to increase patient contact and intervention time?	Excellent points. We now discuss these points in the results and limitations. We don't know how these interventions would work for other conditions, but we now point out some unique characteristics of depression that might predict more impact for this condition than others. We also point out why, while they are characteristic of any good treatment plan, they are particularly difficult to achieve for depression in primary care. The effect of lowering panel size and increasing time with primary care would be an excellent thing to study; it might, however, be considerably more costly than adding staff for care management (so I was told by Kaiser upper management when it was proposed during my quality improvement study there).
Results	No indication of cvert bias; much potential for subjective bias in this study during abstraction of variables (eg. last paragraph, page 18)	
Results	Page 24 Qualitative Analysis of Intervention Features vs Outcome Impacts: "These were all commonly used so it is hard to say how critical they really are"	Changed language. Basically, we know the features characterized most of the sample of studies, which overall were effective, and we also know they clustered in the most impactful studies. But we don't know that taking any one of them out would undo the effect. Still can say that to mirror the literature, people should adhere to these features, pending additional information.
Results	.[With respect to following Report statement on page 25: No study excluded anxiety. Six studies (21%) did not mention PTSD, and only 14% of the remaining 22 studies excluded patients based on it. Six studies (21%) did not report on the proportion of minorities enrolled.] "Alcohol is also not mentioned in these but very common in practice. I would say more that we know these anxiety disorders, cognition, alcohol use, etc are common and we don't know the impact on care management"	Added.
Tables - 1	Significant typo at the bottom of page 27--change "diabetes" to "depression"	Changed.
Tables - 6	Table 6 shows studies that all have the same category of supportive interventions. Many have "yes" responses but then are rated anywhere from 1-4 on impact. The study indicates this was a personal review which had a high level of concurrence in rating. Would it have been better to establish some point values which related to the 1-4 level of ratings rather than enter subjective bias into the review?	Explanations were unclear. We have now included much more information on the impact rating, how it worked, and why it was used in Methods and in Results.

REFERENCES

(2005). Cochrane handbook for systematic reviews of interventions 4.2.5 [updated May 2005]. The Cochrane Library. J. G. Higgins, S. Chichester, UK, 7 John Wiley and Sons: 187-8.

Adler, D. A., K. M. Bungay, et al. (2004). "The impact of a pharmacist intervention on 6-month outcomes in depressed primary care patients." Gen Hosp Psychiatry 26(3): 199-209.

Agency for Health Care Policy and Research (1993). Clinical Practice Guideline: Quick Reference Guide for Clinicians, AHCPR Publication No. 93-0552.

Araya, R., G. Rojas, et al. (2003). "Treating depression in primary care in low-income women in Santiago, Chile: a randomised controlled trial." Lancet 361(9362): 995-1000.

Bartels, S. J., E. H. Coakley, et al. (2004). "Improving access to geriatric mental health services: a randomized trial comparing treatment engagement with integrated versus enhanced referral care for depression, anxiety, and at-risk alcohol use." Am J Psychiatry 161(8): 1455-62.

Berkey, C. S., D. C. Hoaglin, et al. (1995). "A random-effects regression model for meta-analysis." Stat Med 14(4): 395-411.

Bodenheimer, T., E. H. Wagner, et al. (2002). "Improving primary care for patients with chronic illness." JAMA 288(14): 1775-9.

Bodenheimer, T., E. H. Wagner, et al. (2002). "Improving primary care for patients with chronic illness: the chronic care model, Part 2." JAMA 288(15): 1909-14.

Bower, P. and B. Sibbald (2000). "On-site mental health workers in primary care: effects on professional practice." Cochrane Database Syst Rev(3): CD000532.

Brook, O. H., H. van Hout, et al. (2005). "A pharmacy-based coaching program to improve adherence to antidepressant treatment among primary care patients." Psychiatr Serv 56(4): 487-9.

Bruce, M. L., T. R. Ten Have, et al. (2004). "Reducing suicidal ideation and depressive symptoms in depressed older primary care patients: a randomized controlled trial." JAMA 291(9): 1081-91.

Butler, M., R.L. Kane, et al. (2008). Integration of Mental Health/Substance Abuse and Primary Care. AHRQ Publication No. 09-E003, Oct. Available at http://www.ahrq.gov/clinic/tp/mhsapctp.htm. Accessed 1/09.

Capoccia, K. L., D. M. Boudreau, et al. (2004). "Randomized trial of pharmacist interventions to improve depression care and outcomes in primary care." Am J Health Syst Pharm 61(4): 364-72.

Craven, M. A. and R. Bland (2002). "Shared mental health care: a bibliography and overview." Can J Psychiatry 47(2 Suppl 1): iS-viiiS, 1S-103S.

Craven, M. A. and R. Bland (2006). "Better practices in collaborative mental health care: an analysis of the evidence base." Can J Psychiatry 51(6 Suppl 1): 7S-72S.

Datto, C. J., R. Thompson, et al. (2003). "The pilot study of a telephone disease management program for depression." Gen Hosp Psychiatry 25(3): 169-77.

Dietrich, A. J., T. E. Oxman, et al. (2004). "Re-engineering systems for the treatment of depression in primary care: cluster randomised controlled trial." BMJ 329(7466): 602.

Dobscha, S. K., K. Corson, et al. (2006). "Depression decision support in primary care: a cluster randomized trial." Ann Intern Med 145(7): 477-87.

Finley, P. R., H. R. Rens, et al. (2003). "Impact of a collaborative care model on depression in a primary care setting: a randomized controlled trial." Pharmacotherapy 23(9): 1175-85.

Fortney, J. C., et al (2006). Telemedicine-based collaborative care to reduce rural disparities. Health Services Research and Development Meeting. Washignton, DC.

Gilbody, S., P. Bower, et al. (2006). "Collaborative care for depression: a cumulative meta-analysis and review of longer-term outcomes." Arch Intern Med 166(21): 2314-21.

Gilbody, S., P. Bower, et al. (2006). "Costs and consequences of enhanced primary care for depression: systematic review of randomised economic evaluations." Br J Psychiatry 189: 297-308.

Gilbody, S., P. Whitty, et al. (2003). "Educational and organizational interventions to improve the management of depression in primary care: a systematic review." JAMA 289(23): 3145-51.

Goldberg, D. P., J. J. Steele, et al. (1980). "Training family doctors to recognize psychiatric illness with increased accuracy." Lancer: 521-523.

Hedrick, S. C., E. F. Chaney, et al. (2003). "Effectiveness of collaborative care depression treatment in Veterans' Affairs primary care." J Gen Intern Med 18(1): 9-16.

Hepner, K. A., M. Rowe, et al. (2007). "The effect of adherence to practice guidelines on depression outcomes." Ann Intern Med 147(5): 320-9.

Higgins, J. and S. Green Approaches to summarizing the validity of studies. Cochrane Handbook for Systematic Reviews of Interventions 4.2.5 [updated May 2005]; Section 6.7. In: the Cochrane Library, Issue 3, 2005. Chichester, UK, John Wiley & Sons.

Hunkeler, E. M., J. F. Meresman, et al. (2000). "Efficacy of nurse telehealth care and peer support in augmenting treatment of depression in primary care." Arch Fam Med 9(8): 700-8.

IMPACT Implementation Center (2008). Tools and Materials for Depression Care. Available at: http://www.rand.org/health/surveys_tools/pic.htm. Accessed 1/09.

Institute of Medicine (2001). Crossing the Quality Chasm : A New Health System for the 21st Century. Washington, National Academy Press.

Katon, W. (1995). "Collaborative care: patient satisfaction, outcomes, and medical cost-offset." Fam Syst Med 13(3-4): 351-65.

Katon, W., P. Robinson, ct al. (1996). "A multifaceted intervention to improve treatment of depression in primary care." Arch Gen Psychiatry 53(10): 924-32.

Katon, W., C. Rutter, et al. (2001). "A randomized trial of relapse prevention of depression in primary care." Arch Gen Psychiatry 58(3): 241-7.

Katon, W. and H. Schulberg (1992). "Epidemiology of depression in primary care." Gen Hosp Psychiatry 14(4): 237-47.

Katon, W., M. von Korff, et al. (1992). "Adequacy and duration of antidepressant treatment in primary care." Med Care 30(1): 67-76.

Katon, W., M. Von Korff, et al. (2001). "Rethinking practitioner roles in chronic illness: the specialist, primary care physician, and the practice nurse." Gen Hosp Psychiatry 23(3): 138-44.

Katon, W., M. Von Korff, et al. (1999). "Stepped collaborative care for primary care patients with persistent symptoms of depression: a randomized trial." Arch Gen Psychiatry 56(12): 1109-15.

Katon, W., M. Von Korff, et al. (1995). "Collaborative management to achieve treatment guidelines. Impact on depression in primary care." JAMA 273(13): 1026-31.

Katon, W. J., M. Von Korff, et al. (1995). "Collaborative management to achieve treatment guidelines: Impact on depression in primary care." Journal of American Medical Association 273(13): 1026-1031.

Katon, W. J., M. Von Korff, et al. (2004). "The Pathways Study: a randomized trial of collaborative care in patients with diabetes and depression." Arch Gen Psychiatry 61(10): 1042-9.

Katzelnick, D. J., G. E. Simon, et al. (2000). "Randomized trial of a depression management program in high utilizers of medical care." Arch Fam Med 9(4): 345-51.

Lin, E. H., W. J. Katon, et al. (2000). "Low-intensity treatment of depression in primary care: is it problematic?" Gen Hosp Psychiatry 22(2): 78-83.

Lo Sasso, A. T., K. Rost, et al. (2006). "Modeling the impact of enhanced depression treatment on workplace functioning and costs: a cost-benefit approach." Med Care 44(4): 352-8.

Macarthur Foundation (2003). Depression in Primary Care Tools and Materials. Chicago, IL, John D. and Catherine T. MacAuthur Foundation. Available at http://depression-primary-care.org/ . Accessed 1/09.

Mann, A. H., R. Blizard, et al. (1998). "An evaluation of practice nurses working with general practitioners to treat people with depression." Br J Gen Pract 48(426): 875-9.

Miles, M. B. and A. M. Huberman (1994). Qualitative Data Analysis: A source book for new methods. Thousand Oaks, Sage Publications.

Mitchell, G., C. Del Mar, et al. (2002). "Does primary medical practitioner involvement with a specialist team improve patient outcomes? A systematic review." Br J Gen Pract 52(484): 934-9.

Murray, C. J. and A. D. Lopez (1997). "Alternative projections of mortality and disability by cause 1990-2020: Global Burden of Disease Study." Lancet 349(9064): 1498-504.

Ormel J, V. M., Ustun TB, Pini S, Korten A, Oldehinkel T (1994). "Common mental disorders and disability across cultures. Results from the WHO Collaborative Study on Psychological Problems in General Health Care." JAMA 272: 1741-8.

Oslin, D. W., S. Sayers, et al. (2003). "Disease management for depression and at-risk drinking via telephone in an older population of veterans." Psychosom Med 65(6): 931-7.

Oxman, T. E., A. J. Dietrich, et al. (2002). "A three-component model for reengineering systems for the treatment of depression in primary care." Psychosomatics 43(6): 441-50.

Peveler, R., C. George, et al. (1999). "Effect of antidepressant drug counselling and information leaflets on adherence to drug treatment in primary care: randomised controlled trial." BMJ 319(7210): 612-5.

RAND (2000). Partners in Care Tools and Materials. Available at: http://www.rand.org/health/surveys_tools/pic.htm. Accessed 1/09.

Rickles, N. M., B. L. Svarstad, et al. (2005). "Pharmacist telemonitoring of antidepressant use: effects on pharmacist-patient collaboration." J Am Pharm Assoc (2003) 45(3): 344-53.

Robinson, K. A. and K. Dickersin (2002). "Development of a highly sensitive search strategy for the retrieval of reports of controlled trials using PubMed." Int J Epidemiol 31(1): 150-3.

Rollman, B. L., B. H. Hanusa, et al. (2002). "A randomized trial using computerized decision support to improve treatment of major depression in primary care." J Gen Intern Med 17(7): 493-503.

Rost, K., P. Nutting, et al. (2001). "Improving depression outcomes in community primary care practice: a randomized trial of the quEST intervention. Quality Enhancement by Strategic Teaming." J Gen Intern Med 16(3): 143-9.

Rubenstein, L. V., D. R. Calkins, et al. (1989). "Improving patient function: A randomized trial of functional disability screening." Annals of Internal Medicine 111: 836-842.

Rubenstein, L. V., J. M. McCoy, et al. (1995). "Improving patient quality of life with feedback to physicians about functional status." J Gen Intern Med 10(11): 607-14.

Rubenstein, L. V., L. S. Meredith, et al. (2006). "Impacts of evidence-based quality improvement on depression in primary care: a randomized experiment." J Gen Intern Med. 21(10): 1027-35. Epub 2006 Jul 7.

Rubenstein, L. V., L. E. Parker, et al. (2002). "Understanding team-based quality improvement for depression in primary care." Health Serv Res 37(4): 1009-29.

Schoenbaum, M., C. Sherbourne, et al. (2005). "Gender patterns in cost effectiveness of quality improvement for depression: results of a randomized, controlled trial." J Affect Disord 87(2-3): 319-25.

Schoenbaum, M., J. Unutzer, et al. (2002). "The effects of primary care depression treatment on patients' clinical status and employment." Health Serv Res 37(5): 1145-58.

Simon, G. E., E. J. Ludman, et al. (2004). "Telephone psychotherapy and telephone care management for primary care patients starting antidepressant treatment: a randomized controlled trial." JAMA 292(8): 935-42.

Simon, G. E. and M. VonKorff (1995). "Recognition, management, and outcomes of depression in primary care." Arch Fam Med 4(2): 99-105.

Simon, G. E., M. VonKorff, et al. (2000). "Randomised trial of monitoring, feedback, and management of care by telephone to improve treatment of depression in primary care." BMJ 320(7234): 550-4.

Stata (2006). Statistical Software Manual. College Station, TX, Stata Corp.

Stone, E. G., S. C. Morton, et al. (2002). "Interventions that increase use of adult immunization and cancer screening services: a meta-analysis." Ann Intern Med 136(9): 641-51.

Sutton AJ, A. K., Jones DR, Sheldon TR, Song F (2000). "Methods for Meta-Analysis in Medical Research." Wiley: 29-31.

Swindle, R. W., J. K. Rao, et al. (2003). "Integrating clinical nurse specialists into the treatment of primary care patients with depression." Int J Psychiatry Med 33(1): 17-37.

Thompson, C., A. L. Kinmonth, et al. (2000). "Effects of a clinical-practice guideline and practice-based education on detection and outcome of depression in primary care: Hampshire Depression Project randomised controlled trial." Lancet 355(9199): 185-91.

Unutzer, J., W. Katon, et al. (2002). "Collaborative care management of late-life depression in the primary care setting: a randomized controlled trial." JAMA 288(22): 2836-45.

Von Korff, M., J. Gruman, et al. (1997). "Collaborative management of chronic illness." Annals of Internal Medicine 127(12): 1097-102.

Wagner, E. H., B. T. Austin, et al. (2001). "Improving chronic illness care: translating evidence into action." Health Aff (Millwood) 20(6): 64-78.

Wagner, E. H., B. T. Austin, et al. (2001). "Improving chronic illness care: translating evidence into action." Health Aff (Millwood) 20(6): 64-78.

Wagner, E. H., R. E. Glasgow, et al. (2001). "Quality Improvement In Chronic Illness Care: A Collaborative Approach." Joint Commission Journal on Quality Improvement 27(2): 63-80.

Waterreus, A., M. Blanchard, et al. (1994). "Community psychiatric nurses for the elderly: well tolerated, few side-effects and effective in the treatment of depression." J Clin Nurs 3(5): 299-306.

Wells, K. B., C. Sherbourne, et al. (2000). "Impact of disseminating quality improvement programs for depression in managed primary care: a randomized controlled trial." JAMA 283(2): 212-20.

Wells, K., C. Sherbourne, et al. (2005). "Quality improvement for depression in primary care: do patients with subthreshold depression benefit in the long run?" Am J Psychiatry 162(6): 1149-57.

Williams, J. W., Jr., M. Gerrity, et al. (2007). "Systematic review of multifaceted interventions to improve depression care." Gen Hosp Psychiatry 29(2): 91-116.

Zhang, M., K. M. Rost, et al. (1999). "A community study of depression treatment and employment earnings." Psychiatr Serv 50(9): 1209-13.